Transformative Community Health Nursing

Sakiko Kanbara
Editor

Transformative Community Health Nursing

Open Governance and Disaster Resilience in the Digital Age

Springer

Editor
Sakiko Kanbara
Kobe City College of Nursing
Kobe, Hyogo, Japan

ISBN 978-3-032-24404-8 ISBN 978-3-032-24405-5 (eBook)
https://doi.org/10.1007/978-3-032-24405-5

This Springer imprint is published by the registered company Springer Nature Switzerland AG
The registered company address is: Gewerbestrasse 11, 6330 Cham, Switzerland

Preface

The world stands at a threshold. Climate crises intensify, pandemics spread across digital and physical networks, demographic shifts hollow rural communities while overwhelming urban centers, and digital disruption reshapes how we communicate, work, and care for one another.

In 2015, three foundational international commitments converged to reframe how the world understands health, risk, and governance:

- The UN Sustainable Development Goals (SDGs), with their cross-cutting imperative to leave no one behind
- The Sendai Framework for Disaster Risk Reduction (2015–2030): a global commitment to understanding disaster not as inevitable fate but as a series of preventable and manageable risks that societies can collectively reduce
- The WHO Integrated People-Centred Health Services (IPCHS) Strategy: a vision of health systems designed around the needs, preferences, and agency of people, not institutions

Together, these frameworks called for a fundamental shift—one that nursing is uniquely positioned to lead.

Over the past decades, nursing has evolved significantly in its understanding of disaster response. Yet the profession has often remained within familiar silos: responding to acute crises, managing hospitals, and implementing top-down public health programs.

But disasters no longer fit neat emergency categories. A flood cascades into disease outbreaks, food insecurity, and psychological trauma. A pandemic becomes simultaneously a health crisis, an economic catastrophe, and a moment of profound social fragmentation. Climate change transforms these patterns into permanent conditions of risk. These are not isolated crises—they are cascading, interconnected risks that expose the deepest vulnerabilities in our health systems and societies: persistent inequities, fragmented governance, and the absence of meaningful community voice in decisions that affect survival itself.

Simultaneously, a counter-movement has emerged. In Japan and globally, communities are discovering their own agency. Citizens are not waiting for government or experts; they are mapping their own risks, caring for their neighbors, organizing mutual aid networks, and demanding a voice in the governance of their own resilience. This book documents and amplifies that movement.

In this moment of systemic fragility, this book poses a provocative claim: nursing must be transformed—from a profession primarily defined by clinical care to a driver of social innovation and open governance. The largest and most trusted health profession in the world, nursing is uniquely positioned to bridge policy, technology, and community action in ways that generate sustainable resilience.

Transformative Community Health Nursing emerges from a distinctive collaborative process from Japan and across the globe. Jimoto—places with deep roots and living memory—devastated by disaster became laboratories for innovative, equitable, and participatory health systems.

The Three Pillars: An Integrated Framework

This volume rests on the integration of three traditionally separate domains:

1. Disaster Nursing: Historically focused on emergency response, disaster nursing is being redefined as a systems-level discipline concerned with proactive resilience, social cohesion, and the long-term capacity of communities to anticipate, withstand, and recover from shocks. Beyond triage and first aid, disaster nursing now encompasses disaster literacy, community preparedness, governance structures, and the protection of vulnerable populations before crisis strikes.
2. Primary Health Care (PHC): The WHO's foundational commitment to health equity and community-centered care has never been more urgent. This book interprets PHC not as a set of isolated programs but as a foundation for systemic transformation. Central to this vision is the concept of Jimoto Sousei Nursing, in Japan—Local Social Innovation as Primary Health Care—which frames nursing as a catalyst for place-based, community-led solutions grounded in local culture, knowledge, and resources.
3. Digital Transformation: Technology is not neutral. When designed with community input and accountable governance, digital systems can amplify human connection, democratize information, and enable rapid, adaptive responses to cascading risks. When imposed top-down without community voice, the same technologies deepen divides and marginalize the most vulnerable. This book navigates that tension: how can nursing harness Society 5.0 technologies in service of equity and human dignity?

Nursing, uniquely, has the capacity to embody and champion all three. Throughout this book, these pillars become concrete through empirical cases, community voices, and practical tools.

The Bold Claim at the Heart of This Book

The fundamental argument is this: Sustainable resilience requires more than technology, infrastructure, or policy mandates. It requires care, equity, and participatory governance. Care—the commitment to tend to the whole person, to recognize dignity and interdependence, to honor the will to live—is not sentiment. It is the foundation of trust without which no community can organize for collective action. Equity—the systematic removal of barriers that condemn some to vulnerability while insulating others from risk—is not charity. It is a recognition that all lives have equal moral worth and that societies that tolerate preventable suffering corrode from within. Participatory governance—the insistence that those affected by decisions must have voice in making them—is not inefficient. It is the only pathway to policies and systems that are simultaneously legitimate, effective, and sustainable.

Who This Book Is For

This volume is written for community health nurses and public health practitioners, Advanced Practice Nurses positioned to lead systems change, disaster management professionals, policymakers and government officials, nursing educators and scholars, students across nursing and adjacent fields, and community leaders seeking to understand how health professionals can become allies in community-led resilience.

Acknowledgments

This book would not exist without the people who made its knowledge possible—not only as research subjects, but as co-creators, teachers, and partners.

To Professor Hiroko Minami, whose visionary leadership has guided the Disaster Nursing Global Leadership program and continued to elevate disaster nursing as a discipline worthy of the world's most urgent challenges: your mentorship, integrity, and unwavering commitment to the profession have been a constant source of inspiration and strength.

To the citizens of Kochi who welcomed us into their communities, shared their lives and worries, and showed us what it means to build resilience from the ground up: this book is, in many ways, yours. Your willingness to experiment, to speak honestly about what works and what does not, and to keep showing up has shaped every page.

To the survivors of the 2018 Western Japan Floods in Kurashiki-Mabi—my hometown—who found the strength to care for one another even in the midst of devastating loss: you demonstrated, more powerfully than any framework could, that community is not a concept but a living practice of mutual obligation.

We offer this book with deep humility. It is not a theoretical treatise, but a living record of practice in evolution—documenting the insights, frameworks, and practical tools that have emerged from on-the-ground experience and rigorous scholarship. At its core, this book is a love letter to the nursing profession—and a challenge: nursing has always been about service, compassion, and the protection of the vulnerable. Now it must become something more: a force for systemic transformation toward a world where all communities have the power to author their own resilience.

Kobe, Japan Sakiko Kanbara

Contents

Editor and Contributors

About the Editor

Sakiko Kanbara is a Professor in the Faculty of Nursing at Kobe City College of Nursing, Japan. She is currently a Member of the Science Council of Japan, a Board Member of the AI Disaster Prevention Council, and serves as a Judge for the Challenge Open Governance initiative in Japan. She received her BS and MS in Health Science from Kobe University and her PhD from Okayama University.From 2006, she served as an Investigator at the Centre of Excellence for Disaster Nursing in Ubiquitous Society, Research Institute of Nursing Care for People and Community, WHO Collaboration Centre for Nursing in Disaster and Health Emergency, University of Hyogo. In 2012, she joined the University of Kochi as Associate Professor and subsequently Professor (from 2018) of the Doctoral Degree Program for Disaster Nursing Global Leadership (DNGL), funded by the Ministry of Education, Culture, Sports, Science and Technology (MEXT), Japan.During her tenure at the University of Kochi, she responded to Typhoon Haiyan (2013) and the Nepal Earthquake (2015), and in 2015 founded EpiNurse, a social enterprise advancing community-based disaster health management. She also launched the Gensai Care Project (Disaster Mitigation Care Project), a participatory research initiative linking primary health care with community resilience. Following the 2018 Western Japan Floods, she led multiple projects in the affected Kurashiki-Mabi district—her hometown—including the development of the Participatory Caring Map, a community-driven open data initiative.Her work and collaborative projects have been recognized internationally with multiple awards, including the Risk Award at the 2017 Global Platform for Disaster Risk Reduction, the Special Innovation Award (2019) from the Ash Center for Democratic Governance and Innovation, Harvard Kennedy School, the Excellence Award at the Ministry of Internal Affairs and Communications (MIC) ICT Regional Revitalization Grand Prize (2020), and the Interspace Collaboration Research Center Award at the WIRED Common Ground Challenge (2022), among others.In 2024, she chaired the 8th World Society of Disaster Nursing Conference in Kobe, advancing global collaboration in disaster risk reduction, themed "Rethinking Disaster Nursing in the Changing Risk Landscape: From Primary Health Care to Social Innovation for Planetary Health."

Contributors

Megumi Fujii Faculty of Nursing, Japanese Red Cross Toyota College of Nursing, Toyota, Japan

Noriko Hatakeyama Faculty of Health Care and Nursing, Juntendo University, Tokyo, Japan

Yuri Machida Social Design Department, Peace Winds Japan, Kochi, Japan

Sayumi Nojima University of Kochi, Kochi, Japan

Sushila Paudel Faculty of Nursing, University of Kochi, Kochi, Japan

Takashi Naruse Health Care, Wellbeing Research Department, Sompo Institute Plus Inc, Tokyo, Japan

Abbreviations[1]

AI	Artificial Intelligence
API	Application Programming Interface
APN	Advanced Practice Nurse
AX	Augmented Reality
CAP	Community as Partner
CBPR	Community-Based Participatory Research
CCHS	Care-Centered Human Security
COG	Challenge Open Governance
COPD	Chronic Obstructive Pulmonary Disease
COVID-19	Coronavirus Disease 2019
DEI	Diversity, Equity, and Inclusion
DNGL	Disaster Nursing Global Leader initiative
DRR	Disaster Risk Reduction
DX	Digital Transformation
EHR	Electronic Health Record
GDP	Gross Domestic Product
GIS	Geographic Information System
GPS	Global Positioning System
HCD	Human-Centered Design
HEDRM	Health Emergency and Disaster Risk Management
HIV/AIDS	Human Immunodeficiency Virus/Acquired Immunodeficiency Syndrome
ICN	International Council of Nurses
ICT	Information and Communication Technologies
IDNDR	International Decade for Natural Disaster Reduction
ILO	International Labor Organization
IOM	International Organization for Migration
IoT	Internet of Technology
IPCHS	Integrated People-Centered Health Services
ISA	Immigration Services Agency
JMA	Japan Meteorological Agency
LGBTQ	Lesbian, Gay, Bisexual, Transgender, and Queer

[1] The following abbreviations are used throughout this book.

METI	Ministry of Economy, Trade and Industry
MHLW	Ministry of Health, Labor and Welfare
MIC	Ministry of Internal Affairs and Communications
NATECH	Natural Hazards Triggering Technological Disaster
NCDs	Non-Communicable Disease
NGO	Non-Governmental Organization
NIPSSR	National Institute of Population and Social Security Research
OECD	Organization for Economic Co-operation and Development
OHCHR	Office of the High Commissioner for Human Rights
OODA	Observe, Orient, Decide, Act
OSM	OpenStreetMap
PHC	Primary Health Care
PHNs	Public Health Nurses
PHR	Personal Health Record
PICRAT	Passive, Interactive, Creative, Replace, Amplify, Transform
QR	Quick Response (Code)
RACI	Responsible, Accountable, Consulted, Informed
SCJ	Science Council of Japan
SDGs	Sustainable Development Goals
SNS	Social Networking Service
SOAP	Subjective, Objective, Assessment, Plan
SVI	Syndemic Vulnerability Index
TTM	Transtheoretical Model
UHC	Universal Health Coverage
UN	United Nations
UNDP	United Nations Development Programme
UNDRR	United Nations Office for Disaster Risk Reduction
UNHCR	United Nations High Commissioner for Refugees
UNISDR	United Nations International Strategy for Disaster Reduction
VR	Virtual Reality
WHO	World Health Organization
XR	Extended Reality

Redefining Nursing in an Age of Planetary Risk and Human Security: From Nightingale to Digital Transformation—Caring for Health Security and Disaster Resilience

1

Sakiko Kanbara and Sayumi Nojima

1.1 Introduction

The 2020s have shown that health risk is increasingly "compound": a heatwave, a flood, a respiratory outbreak, and the quiet burden of chronic disease can converge in the same community—often affecting the same people. In such moments, what determines outcomes is not only clinical treatment but also whether everyday care systems can remain continuous, inclusive, and trustworthy when infrastructure, information flows, and social networks are strained. This is why nursing must be reconsidered not only as bedside practice but also as a form of care infrastructure that protects dignity and sustains life conditions across homes, communities, shelters, and health services.

This book explores that shift through a Japan-based, globally informed lens. By linking disaster risk reduction (DRR) with primary health care and people-centered governance, it asks how nursing can move from a reactive role to a proactive one—from responding to crisis to designing conditions for resilience. While human security frameworks emphasize protection, resilience, and institutional preparedness, they often under-specify the governance role of social reproduction—the everyday processes that sustain dignity, health, and societal continuity. What remains insufficiently operationalized is not technology, nor policy ambition but the institutional recognition of care as foundational infrastructure. This book, therefore, proceeds from what may tentatively be termed a Care-Centered Human Security Framework (CCHS)—an approach that conceptualizes care not as charity or sectoral service but

S. Kanbara (✉)
Faculty of Nursing, Kobe City College of Nursing, Kobe, Japan
e-mail: s-kanbara@kobe-ccn.ac.jp

S. Nojima
University of Kochi, Kochi, Japan
e-mail: nojimas@cc.u-kochi.ac.jp

S. Kanbara (ed.), *Transformative Community Health Nursing*,
https://doi.org/10.1007/978-3-032-24405-5_1

as an operational governance interface linking social policy commitments, institutional coordination between health security and disaster resilience, and accountable data systems. By repositioning care as invisible infrastructure, CCHS seeks to render measurable and governable what has long remained structurally indispensable yet politically peripheral.

This chapter sets the foundation by introducing the lenses of syndemics, planetary health, and human security and by clarifying how they reframe the mission of nursing in an era of global risk.

The challenges facing twenty-first-century nursing are unprecedented in their complexity and scale. Climate change-related disasters have increased by 50% since 2000, disproportionately affecting low-income countries (UNDRR, 2021). Meanwhile, pandemic threats loom large, with the WHO estimating that the world faces at least one major infectious disease outbreak per year (WHO, 2023). Against this backdrop, the nursing workforce—comprising over 28 million practitioners globally—represents the largest segment of healthcare providers and the most trusted profession in most countries (Gallup, 2020). Yet this workforce remains underutilized in policymaking and disaster governance, despite nurses constituting the majority of frontline responders (ICN, 2019). This chapter argues that elevating nursing from a reactive to a proactive role—from care providers to system designers—is essential for achieving health security in an era of compounding risks. To help readers navigate the many concepts introduced, this chapter is structured around three functions:

- *What (Definitions)*: We clarify the three key lenses—*Syndemic, Planetary Health, and Human Security*—and how they overlap.
- *Why (Rationale)*: We ground the urgency in global frameworks (Sustainable Development Goals [SDGs], Sendai Framework, WHO strategies) and the realities of health inequity and compounded risks.
- *How (Implementation)*: We translate risk models into nursing actions, propose practice roles and evaluation indicators, and highlight ethics and governance for data-informed care.

1.1.1 What: A Three-Lens Framework

Human Security (Centering Dignity): A paradigm shift from national defense to people-centered protection. It safeguards the "vital core" of all human lives—freedom from fear, freedom from want, and freedom to live in dignity—especially during crises (Commission on Human Security, 2003; UNDP, 1994).
Syndemic (Contextualizing Risk): Beyond isolated epidemics, this lens reveals how disease concentrations (e.g., COVID-19, NCDs) interact with social, environmental, and economic inequities to amplify vulnerability (Mendenhall, 2017).

Global Nursing Implication: Nurses must treat the "synergy of epidemics" by addressing the root causes of inequality, not just the biological symptoms.

Planetary Health (Expanding Scope): A transdisciplinary framework emphasizing that human health is inseparable from the natural systems of the Earth. It positions the planet's stability as the ultimate determinant of health (Horton et al., 2014).

Global Nursing Implication: Stewardship extends from the bedside to the biosphere; climate action and environmental advocacy are now fundamental components of nursing care. In disasters and conflict, nurses act as the primary agents of human security, protecting the most vulnerable when systems fail.

Modern nursing, as initiated by Nightingale, was fundamentally about restoring order, dignity, and safety amid chaos. By focusing on "clean air and water" and efficient management, she demonstrated that health is intrinsically linked to our living and working environments. Even in the absence of advanced medicine, her environmental interventions saved lives (Nightingale, 1860). Her most enduring contribution was not only bedside compassion but also the conviction that *health is shaped by environment and governance*. Nightingale's interventions—ventilation, sanitation, clean water, and efficient management—demonstrated that lives can be saved even without advanced medicine when daily living conditions are improved. In that sense, nursing began as a form of *social design*: restoring order, dignity, and safety amid chaos.

1.1.2 Why: Global Risk Landscape and Health Inequity

Multiple, interacting risks define today's health landscape. Pandemics, climate-related disasters, urbanization, population aging, chronic disease, and widening inequities no longer arrive as separate events—they compound across time and place. This is what is increasingly described as a *syndemic*: a synergistic clustering of epidemics shaped by social, environmental, and economic conditions (Mendenhall et al., 2022). The common disaster risk formula—Risk = Hazard × Vulnerability/Capacity (Wisner et al., 2004)—makes this tractable for nursing practice. Rapid population aging and urbanization increase vulnerability, while environmental degradation erodes a community's capacity to cope. This equation is often presented as a technical tool. For nursing, its value is practical: it clarifies *where nursing can move the variables*. Nurses rarely control hazards (earthquakes, typhoons, and pandemics), but nursing can measurably reduce vulnerability and strengthen capacity—especially when vulnerability is understood as more than medical risk (Table 1.1). Scientific evidence, such as the WHO's *The Solid Facts* (Wilkinson & Marmot, 2003), indicates that health is not simply a matter of genetics or access to medical care but is intrinsically linked to economic and social factors. Worsening natural disasters further exacerbate these health disparities, devastating individuals and families while placing significant strain on welfare budgets and economies (Benson & Clay, 2004).

In real communities, vulnerability appears as follows:

- Limited information access and digital exclusion.
- Social isolation and loss of mutual aid.

Table 1.1 Position nursing within compounded risks (disasters, infectious diseases, climate change, chronic diseases, and social issues) using a "risk type × response model" matrix

Global risk type (hazard domain)	Risk pathway (typical syndemic interaction)	Nursing roles (prevention → preparedness → response → recovery)	Key "variable" nurses influence (vulnerability/capacity)
Climate-related disasters (heat/flood/storm, etc.)	Disaster + displacement + NCDs/mental health	Heat-health support, evacuation planning, shelter health, long-term follow-up	↓Vulnerability (mobility, resources); ↑Capacity (preparedness, networks)
Geophysical disasters (earthquake/tsunami, etc.)	Mass disruption + care collapse	Triage + "care continuity" in shelters/home, coordination across sectors	↑Capacity (continuity, coordination)
Social risks (poverty, discrimination, digital divide, etc.)	Exclusion + mistrust + health deterioration	Advocacy, navigation, culturally safe care, co-creation forums	↓Vulnerability (barriers); ↑Capacity (participation)
Chronic disease burden	NCDs + poverty + service fragmentation	Preventive care, adherence support, community-based monitoring	↓Vulnerability (care gaps); ↑Capacity (self-management)
Infectious threats (e.g., pandemics)	Infection + chronic disease + inequity	Outreach/PHC, infection prevention, trust-building, continuity for frail people	↓Vulnerability (access, isolation); ↑Capacity (self-care, trust)

- Mobility constraints (disability, frailty, transportation).
- Disrupted care resources and supply chains.
- Discrimination, language barriers, and weak trust in institutions. (These "less obvious" determinants are central to why fragmented, hospital-centered systems fail vulnerable populations.)

Capacity, in turn, is not only hospital surge capacity; it includes the following:

- Self-care and health literacy.
- Community networks and preparedness routines.
- Continuity of primary health care and long-term care.
- Governance mechanisms for coordination and accountability.
- Data systems that make invisible needs visible (without violating dignity).

Despite these challenges, traditional health policies in countries like Japan often remain fragmented. The focus on hospital-based, disease-specific treatment models undermines the system's ability to provide universal, equitable, and sustainable care in a "super-aged" society. Service providers need to reach out to the populations they serve, rather than waiting for patients to arrive. As the UN (2020) notes, where

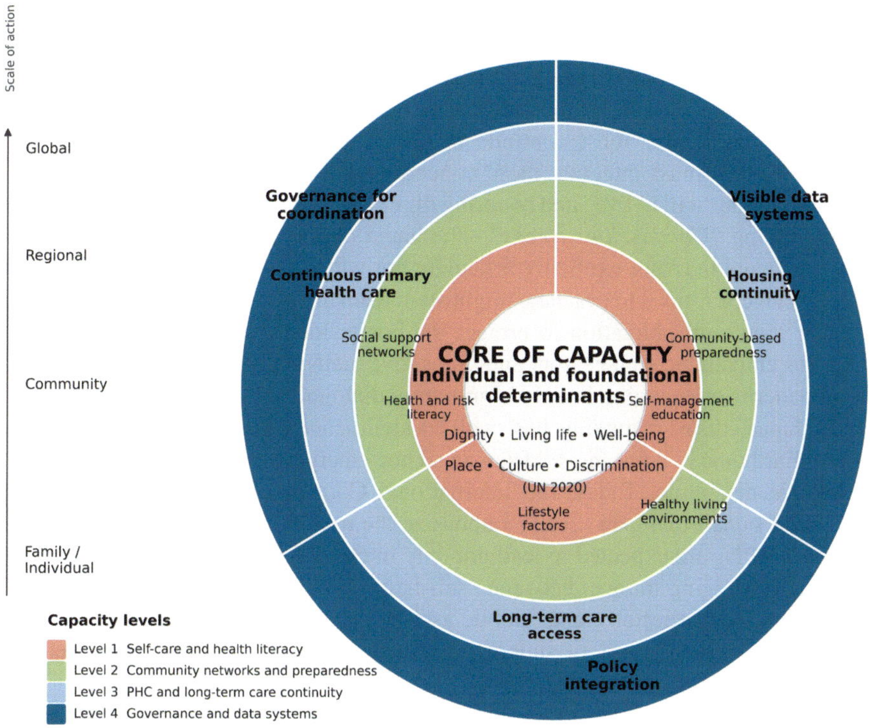

Fig. 1.1 A multi-level framework of health capacity: individual determinants, community networks, and governance across scales of action. (Source: Authors)

people live affects their health status and life opportunities; thus, policies must address less obvious factors such as social support networks, culture, and exposure to discrimination (Fig. 1.1).

1.1.3 How: Global Risk Matrix and Nursing Roles

1.2 Nursing's Role in Strengthening Human Security

To address these vulnerabilities effectively, we must first redefine the core mission of nursing in this era. That mission is Human Security. Nurses operate at the frontline of Human Security, a concept emphasizing the protection of the vital core of all human lives in ways that enhance human freedoms and fulfillment (Commission on Human Security, 2003). From disaster shelters to long-term care facilities, nurses engage with the most intimate, invisible dimensions of vulnerability. This mission requires redefining the dichotomy of "Care" and "Cure." While "cure" focuses on medical treatment to alleviate illness and symptoms, "care" in nursing is deeply connected to Human Security. Care involves protecting the human right to health, maintaining safety, and ensuring access to essentials like clean water, nutrition, and shelter. In times of disaster, hospitals may become dysfunctional due to a lack of resources, but "care" must continue in the community, evacuation centers, and homes. Nurses must integrate these concepts, understanding that "care" is about supporting the "will to live" and restoring dignity. A critical challenge in this domain is addressing "*Unconscious Needs*"—the latent desires, fears, and cultural values that survivors may not explicitly articulate but which strongly influence recovery. For instance, a refusal to evacuate might stem from an unspoken fear of social isolation or a cultural obligation to protect the home. Identifying these hidden needs requires empathetic engagement and innovative methods, such as analyzing behavioral patterns or engaging in deep community dialogue.

In Japan, disaster nursing has evolved significantly since the Great Hanshin-Awaji Earthquake. It has moved from an ad hoc emergency response to a systematic academic discipline. Today, the International Council of Nurses (ICN) and the Science Council of Japan (2011) emphasize the role of Advanced Practice Nurses (APNs). APNs are expected to lead not only in clinical care but also in community advocacy, bridging the gap between "self-help" (individual actions), "mutual aid" (community cooperation), and "public assistance" (government support). By integrating these three layers of support, nurses help build a resilient safety net that withstands shocks.

Human security is not a universal experience but is deeply shaped by cultural contexts, historical trauma, and social identities. What constitutes "security" varies dramatically across cultures. For instance:

In collectivist societies such as many Asian communities, security is often defined in terms of family and community cohesion rather than individual autonomy.

Among Indigenous populations globally, land and environmental stewardship are inseparable from human security, reflecting a worldview where human and planetary health are one (Whyte, 2017).

For refugee and internally displaced populations, security involves both physical safety and the restoration of dignity, cultural practices, and social networks disrupted by conflict or disaster (UNHCR, 2018).

Nurses working in cross-cultural contexts must develop cultural humility—an ongoing commitment to self-reflection and learning about others' cultures without assuming expertise (Tervalon & Murray-García, 1998). This requires the following:

1. *Active Listening*: Creating spaces where marginalized voices can articulate their own definitions of security and needs.
2. *Cultural Brokers*: Partnering with community leaders, traditional healers, and cultural liaisons who understand local meanings of vulnerability and resilience.

3. *Anti-Oppressive Practice*: Recognizing how systems of power (racism, colonialism, and patriarchy) create and perpetuate insecurity and actively working to dismantle these structures.

The concept of “Unconscious Needs” introduced earlier must be understood through this cultural lens. What appears “unconscious” may actually be culturally embedded knowledge that dominant healthcare systems fail to recognize or value. For example, in disaster settings, Western-trained nurses might prioritize individual privacy in evacuation shelters, while survivors from collectivist cultures might derive security from communal living arrangements. Cultural competence in disaster nursing means adapting interventions to honor these differences while ensuring safety.

1.3 The Paradigm Shift: Integrated People-Centered Health Services (IPCHS)

While nurses act as agents of human security, individual efforts are not enough against syndemic risks. To realize human security on a societal scale, the health system itself must undergo a paradigm shift. To address the limitations of fragmented systems, the World Health Organization advocates for Integrated People-Centered Health Services (IPCHS). This strategy envisions a future in which all people have access to coordinated, continuum-of-care health services that meet their life-course needs (WHO, 2015). The IPCHS framework proposes five interdependent strategic objectives to transform health systems:

Empowering and Engaging People: Enabling individuals, families, and communities to take charge of their own health decisions and become active co-producers of health.
Strengthening Governance and Accountability: Creating transparent, inclusive participatory processes where policies are co-developed with community input.
Reorienting Models of Care: Shifting the focus from “cure” in institutional settings to primary and preventive care in the community.
Coordinating Services: Breaking down silos between health, social services, and disaster management to wrap services around people’s multifaceted needs.
Creating an Enabling Environment: Establishing the leadership, financing, and legal frameworks necessary to support these changes.

Treating disasters purely as “emergency response” is insufficient in a world of compounded crises. The Sendai Framework for disaster risk reduction (2015–2030), aligned with SDG 11, reframes disaster reduction not as an isolated task but as a fundamental design requirement for everyday health and welfare systems (United Nations, 2015a, b). For nursing and health policy, this implies that primary health care (PHC), long-term care, and social services must be built to withstand shocks. Specifically, they must be designed for:

Continuity: Ensuring care persists even when infrastructure fails.
Inclusivity: Creating evacuation and shelter standards that protect the most vulnerable.
Participation: Embedding mechanisms for community voice and accountability.
Regeneration: Ensuring recovery reduces future vulnerability ("Build Back Better") rather than merely restoring the status quo.

This "design logic" serves a distinct purpose: it bridges the gap between global governance and the intimate reality of survival. By embedding resilience into the very structure of care, we move beyond technical safety to the protection of dignity and the "vital core" of life. This brings us to the need for new methods of collaboration.

1.4 Practical Implementation Framework for Disaster Nursing in the Age of Planetary Health: A Competency-Based Pathway Toward ICN Level III (Deployable/APN) Practice

Having established the theoretical foundations of Syndemic Risk, Planetary Health, Human Security, and Interprofessional Integrated People-Centered Health Services (IPCHS) in the preceding sections, we now turn to the question of implementation: How do these concepts translate into actionable nursing practice? This volume is written for nurses who are moving beyond basic preparedness and institution-bound response toward advanced, deployable practice. In particular, it is designed as a learning pathway consistent with the International Council of Nurses (ICN) "Core Competencies in Disaster Nursing—Competencies for Nurses involved in Emergency Medical Teams (Level III)," which focuses on nurses prepared to serve on deployable teams, including Emergency Medical Teams (EMTs) (ICN, 2022). To make the chapter operational, this section adopts a competency-based architecture. We use the ICN Level III structure of eight domains as the organizing scaffold, while embedding the three lenses introduced in this chapter (Syndemic, Planetary Health, and Human Security) as cross-cutting perspectives that shape how each domain is interpreted and enacted. This approach also aligns with advanced practice nursing expectations: nurses at this level do not merely "perform tasks" but also lead coordination, safeguard rights and dignity, and translate evidence into system improvement.

1.4.1 Core Competencies for Contemporary Disaster Nursing (ICN Level III Domains) (ICN, 2022)

ICN organizes Level III disaster nursing competencies into eight domains. Below, Table 1.2 maps these domains to the competency expectations for disaster nursing in the age of planetary health, embedding the three lenses introduced in this chapter—Syndemic, Planetary Health, and Human Security—as cross-cutting perspectives.

Table 1.2 Book-to-competency crosswalk (ICN level III domains × Chapters 2–7)

ICN Level III domain	Chapter 2	Chapter 3	Chapter 4	Chapter 5	Chapter 6	Chapter 7
Preparation and planning	○	◎	○	○	◎	○
Communication	◎	○	◎	○	○	◎
Incident management		◎	○	○		◎
Safety and security		○	○		◎	○
Assessment	○	○	◎	◎	◎	○
Intervention	○	○	○	◎	○	○
Recovery	○	○	○	◎	○	◎
Law and ethics	◎	○	○	○	◎	◎

Legend: ◎ = primary focus; ○ = secondary linkage. (Indicative crosswalk; refine as chapter content is finalized)

1.4.2 Operationalizing Level III/APN Disaster Nursing: Toolkit, Evaluation, Ethics, and Adaptation

To translate the Level III/APN competency domains into day-to-day action, this section proposes three complementary instruments used in sequence: the *Syndemic Vulnerability Index (SVI)*, which integrates health, social, environmental, and infrastructure indicators to identify communities facing the most urgent, compounding risks; the *Unconscious Needs Assessment Protocol*, which complements SVI by surfacing the latent fears, values, and barriers that shape real behavior; and the *IPCHS Readiness Checklist*, which assesses whether a locality can maintain integrated, people-centered services during disruption. Together, they create a coherent pathway: make risk and vulnerability visible → co-design acceptable solutions → align services for continuity across home–shelter–facility–hospital.

Implementation is paired with monitoring at three levels—process, outcomes, and equity/ethics—and requires deliberate workforce development through curricula, simulation, mentorship, and refresher training. Digital tools must be treated as a double-edged capability: powerful for coordination but potentially widening inequities unless transparency, accountability, and community partnership are embedded from the outset. Importantly, all frameworks must be adapted to local contexts—low-resource, conflict-affected, rural, and urban—translating global standards into locally legitimate practice.

1.5 Roadmap of This Book: From Global Risk to Local, People-Centered Action

In the face of syndemic risk, planetary disruption, and widening inequities, moving from fragmented services to holistic approaches requires more than technical solutions. It requires care infrastructures that enable participation, trust, and continuity—linking disaster risk reduction with primary health care and people-centered governance. The remainder of this book translates the three lenses introduced in this chapter—syndemics, planetary health, and human security—into practical concepts and case-based learning, grounded in Japan's evolving nursing practice and its implications for global audiences.

Part I (This chapter and Chaps. 2 and 3) establishes the conceptual foundation and situates Japan's nursing transformation within global and local contexts. Chapter 2 examines trends in community health and primary care and reframes community engagement as *Open Community Development*, emphasizing four key "opens"—open governance, open professionalism, open data, and an open mind. It clarifies how public health and community nursing can serve as catalysts for inclusive empowerment in the digital era. Chapter 3 then shifts the lens to Japan's place-based realities and argues that resilient health systems must be built at the level of *jimoto* (home community)—the lived local sphere of everyday relationships, informal care, and mutual aid. It introduces open governance as practical democracy through regional agoras and highlights how *ownership*—the shift from "someone should solve this" to "we will solve it together"—can be cultivated through transdisciplinary collaboration among residents, government, and professionals.

Part II (Chaps. 4, 5 and 6) moves from foundational concepts to pluralistic, participatory practice. Chapter 4 addresses community care in a globalizing society, focusing on cultural competency, trust-building, and equitable access for increasingly diverse populations, including migrants and those facing language or cultural barriers. Chapter 5 presents a rural case that illustrates how rapid aging, geographic constraints, and the digital divide can become determinants of safety and inequity. It examines how intentional digital inclusion—through accessible design, literacy support, and community participation—can strengthen integrated, people-centered services and disaster preparedness. Chapter 6 advances the discussion through the lens of diversity and social inclusion in disaster prevention planning, showing how participation, facilitation, and the visualization of social and institutional networks can make community plans more realistic—especially by engaging those who are often left out of formal decision-making.

Part III (Chaps. 7 and 8) centers on implementation, reflection, and future capacity. Chapter 7 deepens the argument through a data-driven case from Kurashiki, including the author's jimoto experience in Mabi after the 2018 floods. It demonstrates how open data and participatory mapping can support primary health care and disaster risk reduction by turning community knowledge into shared situational awareness and actionable coordination. Finally, Chap. 8 synthesizes the book's insights into a forward-looking agenda for community-regenerating nursing. It articulates the educational and governance capacities needed to cultivate "Society 5.0 Nightingales"—nursing professionals who can connect care, data, and practical democracy to strengthen human security and resilience, locally and globally.

Readers may approach each chapter as a learning module: use its key concepts and cases to identify risks, stakeholders, and decision points, then translate them into a short, place-based "jimoto action plan" for disaster risk reduction (DRR) and primary health care in your own setting. Instructors and practitioners can use the same materials to facilitate seminars or workshops—comparing contexts across chapters and iteratively refining local strategies through dialogue, reflection, and collaboration.

1.6 Conclusion: From Nightingale to Society 5.0

In that sense, nursing began with the premise that nursing is about "putting the patient in the best condition for nature to act upon him." Today, as we face the Anthropocene, we must expand this mission: we must put communities in the best condition for planetary systems to sustain well-being. The concept of **Society 5.0**—a human-centered society that balances economic advancement with the resolution of social problems by a system that highly integrates cyberspace and physical space—provides an opportunity to reimagine this mission. By integrating AI, IoT, and open data with the ethical principles of care, nurses can co-create adaptive, transparent, and resilient health systems. However, technology alone is not the answer. As we will explore in the Kochi case study and other examples throughout this book, success depends on "high-touch" community engagement that respects local wisdom and "unconscious needs" (Kochi Prefecture, 2022). This book is an invitation to that journey. By connecting the "local" with Planetary Health, we will see how nurse-led social innovations are redefining governance. Through disaster mitigation, citizen science, and "whole-of-society" strategies, nursing will lead the way in realizing a new vision of health: one that is not only curative but also regenerative—ensuring safety, dignity, and resilience for all in a digital age.

Acknowledgments The authors thank Seiko Iimura (research assistant, Kobe City College of Nursing) for her dedicated editorial support, literature coordination, and manuscript preparation throughout this chapter. Drafting was partially supported by generative AI writing tools; all content was critically reviewed, revised, and approved by the authors. The authors also acknowledge the global nursing community and the scholars whose foundational work on planetary health, human security, and syndemics informed this conceptual framework.

Author's Note The perspective presented in this chapter is grounded in our ongoing educational and field-based work. While advancing the Disaster Nursing Global Leader (DNGL) initiative under President Hiroko Minami's leadership and through a president's discretionary research grant that catalyzed local implementation in Kochi, we expanded community partnerships and developed participatory, data-informed approaches that connect disaster mitigation with primary health care. The chapters that follow draw on these experiences to explore how nursing can strengthen human security and resilience through open governance, co-creation, and digital transformation.

Author Contributions Conceptualization: Sakiko Kanbara, Sayumi Nojima. Writing—original draft: Sakiko Kanbara. Writing—review and editing: Sayumi Nojima. Editorial and linguistic assistance provided by a research assistant (Seiko Iimura). Literature search and reference management: research assistant (Seiko Iimura). AI-assisted drafting: Generative AI tools were used to support initial structuring and language refinement under the supervision of Sakiko Kanbara.

References

Benson, C., & Clay, E. J. (2004). *Understanding the economic and financial impacts of natural disasters* (No. 4). World Bank Publications.

Commission on Human Security. (2003). *Human security now*. United Nations.

Gallup. (2020). *U.S. ethics rating rise*. https://news.gallup.com/poll/328136/ethics-ratings-rise-medical-workers-teachers.aspx. Accessed 30 Apr 2025.

Horton, R., Beaglehole, R., Bonita, R., Raeburn, J., McKee, M., & Wall, S. (2014). From public to planetary health: A manifesto. *The Lancet, 383*(9920), 847.

International Council of Nursing (ICN). (2019). *Core competencies in disaster nursing*. Version 2.0.

International Council of Nursing (ICN). (2020). *Guidelines on advanced practice nursing*.

International Council of Nurses (ICN). (2022). *Core competencies in disaster nursing: Competencies for nurses involved in emergency medical teams (Level III)*. International Council of Nurses.

Kochi Prefecture. (2022). *Kochi Prefecture Nankai Trough Earthquake Action Plan*. https://www.pref.kochi.lg.jp/doc/2022110700074/file_contents/file_20221171135919_1.pdf. Accessed 30 Apr 2025 (Japanese).

Mendenhall, E. (2017). Syndemics: A new path for global health research. *The Lancet, 389*(10072), 889–891. https://doi.org/10.1016/S0140-6736(17)30602-5. Accessed 30 Apr 2025.

Mendenhall, E., Newfield, T., & Tsai, A. C. (2022). Syndemic theory, methods, and data. *Social Science & Medicine, 295*, 114656.

Nightingale, F. (1860). *Notes on nursing: What it is, and what it is not*. Harrison.

Science Council of Japan. (2011). *Recommendation: toward establishing an advanced practice nurse system – Recommendations based on global standards*. Science Council of Japan.

Tervalon, M., & Murray-García, J. (1998). Cultural humility versus cultural competence: A critical distinction in defining physician training outcomes in multicultural education. *Journal of Health Care for the Poor and Underserved, 9*(2), 117–125. https://doi.org/10.1353/hpu.2010.0233. Accessed 30 Apr 2025.

United Nations. (2015a). *Transforming our world: the 2030 Agenda for Sustainable Development*. United Nations.

United Nations. (2015b). *Sendai framework for disaster risk reduction 2015–2030*. United Nations Office for Disaster Risk Reduction.

United Nations. (2020). *World social report 2020: Inequality in a rapidly changing world*. https://doi.org/10.18356/7f5d0efc-en. Accessed 30 Apr 2025.

United Nations Development Programme (UNDP). (1994). *Human Development Report 1994*. Oxford University Press.

United Nations Disaster Risk Reduction (UNDRR). (2021). *Climate action and disaster risk reduction*. UN.

United Nations High Commissioner for Refugees (UNHCR). (2018). *Global Report 2018*. UN.

Whyte, K. (2017). Indigenous climate change studies: Indigenizing futures, decolonizing the Anthropocene. *English Language Notes, 55*. https://doi.org/10.1215/00138282-55.1-2.153

Wilkinson, R., & Marmot, M. (Eds.). (2003). *Social determinants of health: The solid facts* (2nd ed.). World Health Organization.

Wisner, B., Blaikie, P., Cannon, T., & Davis, I. (2004). *At risk: Natural hazards, people's vulnerability and disasters* (2nd ed.). Routledge.

World Health Organization (WHO). (2015). *WHO global strategy on people-centred and integrated health services: Interim report*. World Health Organization.

World Health Organization (WHO). (2023). *WHO Advisory Committee on Variola Virus Research: Report of the twenty-fourth meeting, Geneva, 29–30 November 2022*. World Health Organization.

2 Addressing Global Nursing Challenges: Strategies for Resilient Community Health

Takashi Naruse

2.1 Introduction

The Future of Nursing 2020–2030: Mapping a Route to Attain Health Equity underscores the pressing need for nurses to focus on the social and structural determinants of health in the coming decade to promote equity (National Academy of Science, Engineering, and Medicine, National Academy of Medicine, 2021). According to a recent report by the International Council of Nurses, achieving the United Nations' Sustainable Development Goals for long-term well-being and survival by 2030 is doubtful without a renewed commitment from global leaders to "ensure that no one is left behind" (Steward, 2022). Health equity entails ensuring that everyone, irrespective of race, ethnicity, gender, sexual orientation, or physical location, has an equal and fair chance to achieve optimal health (Braveman et al., 2017; National Academies of Sciences, Engineering, and Medicine, National Academy of Medicine, 2021). Unfortunately, for numerous individuals worldwide, reaching a state of high health has remained an elusive objective due to its prohibitive cost. Consequently, healthcare inequalities persist, affecting communities from the most impoverished to the most affluent nations. Frequently, challenges to achieving health equity arise from social and structural determinants of health, which can significantly impede progress in this regard.

2.2 Public Health and Crises

Public health is defined as "the science and art of preventing disease, prolonging life and promoting health through the organized efforts and informed choices of society, organizations, public and private, communities and individuals (Winslow, 1920)." The concept of public health encompasses a broad range of activities aimed at

T. Naruse (✉)
Health Care, Wellbeing Research Department, Sompo Institute Plus Inc, Tokyo, Japan

S. Kanbara (ed.), *Transformative Community Health Nursing*,
https://doi.org/10.1007/978-3-032-24405-5_2

promoting and protecting the health of populations (Gatseva, 2011). These activities include disease surveillance, health promotion, environmental health, health policy development, and healthcare access (Winslow, 1920; Institute of Medicine, 1988). Public health professionals work across various sectors, including government agencies, non-profit organizations, academic institutions, and healthcare settings, to address complex health issues and improve population health outcomes (American Public Health Association, 2025). By advocating for policies that prioritize prevention, promote health equity, and foster community partnerships, public health professionals can work toward creating healthier, more resilient societies. In recent years, the field of public health has faced numerous crises and challenges, ranging from infectious disease outbreaks to non-communicable diseases, environmental hazards, and health disparities. The COVID-19 pandemic has highlighted the importance of robust public health infrastructure and preparedness in responding to global health emergencies (Miyah et al., 2022). It has underscored the interconnectedness of health systems and the need for collaborative, evidence-based approaches to address emerging threats to public health. Furthermore, shifting demographic trends, socioeconomic disparities, and rapid urbanization pose additional challenges to public health efforts worldwide. These trends necessitate innovative strategies and interventions to address the evolving health needs of diverse populations. Public health professionals must adapt to changing circumstances, leverage technological advancements, and engage in interdisciplinary collaboration to effectively address emerging health challenges and promote health equity.

2.3 Public Health Nursing and Recent Crises

Public health nursing is a term that was first coined by Lillian Wald, a pioneering nurse and social worker who founded the Henry Street Settlement in New York City in 1893 (Fee & Bu, 2010). The American Public Health Association defined public health nursing as the practice of promoting and protecting the health of populations, and it focuses on improving population health by emphasizing prevention and attending to multiple determinants of health knowledge from nursing, social, and public health sciences (American Public Health Association, 2013). In recent years, the term "community health nursing" has come to include population-based nursing that encompasses communities beyond the public sector. In this chapter, we do not distinguish between the two and uniformly refer to them as public health nursing. Public health nursing employs a variety of interventions, ranging from individual and family health education to community-wide initiatives such as vaccination campaigns, health screenings, and the development of policies to address social determinants of health. Public health nursing has a rich history that dates back to the early twentieth century, when nurses began to move out of hospitals and into communities to provide direct care and education. In recent years, public health nursing has been at the forefront of responding to global and local health crises. The COVID-19 pandemic, for example, highlighted the vital role of Public Health Nurses (PHNs) in protecting community health and preventive measures (Hassmiller, 2022). PHNs have also been instrumental in responding to natural disasters, working tirelessly to mitigate health impacts and support recovery efforts.

A key aspect of public health nursing is its emphasis on community involvement. Community involvement is one of the critical elements of successful problem-solving with communities. PHNs work closely with other healthcare professionals, government agencies, non-profit organizations, and community groups to develop and implement effective public health strategies. PHNs play a role in developing collaborative partnerships with various community members to address problems (Kulbok et al., 2012). By building strong partnerships and fostering community involvement, PHNs ensure that health interventions are culturally sensitive, accessible, and tailored to the unique needs of each population. Toward a society ensuring that no one is left behind, the role of PHNs in promoting inclusiveness cannot be understated. As we move forward, the commitment to inclusiveness must be reflected in every aspect of the community system and public health nursing activities. Building an inclusive society is an ongoing process that requires the collective effort of all its members. It is about recognizing and celebrating diversity, ensuring equal opportunities, and working together to overcome challenges.

2.4 The Basic Act on Dementia to Promote an Inclusive Society, Japan

Public health and public health nursing activities are crucial in shaping community interventions. In Japan, there is a growing advocacy for the development of an "Inclusive society" as an ideal community model. This concept emphasizes a society where community members and stakeholders actively engage beyond traditional boundaries, fostering a collaborative environment for all residents to thrive (Ministry of Health, Labour, and Welfare, 2025). The push toward an inclusive society arises from the need to address modern challenges such as social isolation, aging populations, and healthcare disparities. These issues highlight the limitations of traditional health and welfare systems and the necessity for innovative community-based solutions.

The concept of an inclusive society is highlighted in several government policies. In 2023, the Japanese government compiled a bill titled "The Basic Act on Dementia to Promote an Inclusive Society" (Ministry of Health, Labour and Welfare, 2023). The aim of this bill is to enable every citizen of Japan to fully express their individual personalities and capabilities, including those with dementia, and to foster a robust society where people with and without dementia support and respect each other, thus realizing a society of coexistence. The background of this bill is the reality of an increasing dementia population. The bill seeks to enhance the support for individuals with dementia to participate in society and achieve self-realization, aiming to improve their quality of life.

2.5 The Community as Partner (CAP) Model as a Key Strategy for Public Health Nursing Challenge

As public health nursing activities range from diverse crises, the need for community involvement has increased. For social change to be long term and relevant to the needs of a community, it must come from the community members themselves (Laverack, 2006). The Community as Partner (CAP) model is an innovative approach in public health nursing that emphasizes the importance of forming partnerships with community members to address health and social issues effectively (Anderson & McFarlane, 2019). This model facilitates a collaborative process where PHNs and community members work together to identify, assess, and address the unique needs and challenges within their community. By valuing the insights and experiences of community members, the CAP model ensures that interventions are culturally relevant and sustainable.

Figure 2.1 shows the CAP model. PHNs start their activities from assessing the community constructed in one core-system (Residents) and eight sub-systems (shown at the top: Physical environment, Education, Safety and Transportation, Policies and Government, Health and Social societies, Communication, Economics, and Recreation). The results of the assessment will be shared and analyzed with community partners (residents, community groups, and other professional organizations), and simultaneously, interventions for prevention (primary, secondary, and tertiary) will be implemented. The output and outcome of interventions will be reflected in re-assessment. The co-circulation process is the principle of the CAP model. The CAP model helps PHNs evaluate and improve community resilience and potential stressors relative to the community.

The concept of community and its resilience are described as wheels with three surrounding lines (Fig. 2.2). Three lines implement the concept of community resilience. When each line goes broader, the community can provide stronger resilience. The solid line represents its normal line of defense or the level of health the community has reached over time (e.g., immunity rate and usual patterns of coping). The flexible line of defense, depicted as a broken line around the community and its normal line of defense, is a buffer zone representing a dynamic level of health resulting from a temporary response to stressors (e.g., preparedness for natural disasters). Within the community are lines of resistance, internal mechanisms that act to defend against stressors (e.g., dementia-friendly public space and a fee-free clinic for immigrant people).

Again, community involvement is essential in CAP. Community members are empowered to take an active role in shaping their environment. This empowerment is achieved through education, resource sharing, and the establishment of platforms for dialogue and collaboration. By involving residents in decision-making processes, communities can develop solutions that are more attuned to local needs and circumstances. In the field of public health nursing, numerous benefits of involving residents in community decision-making are discussed (Bruce, 2019). Collaborating with community members helps to promote awareness and understanding of community health needs. By involving residents in decision-making processes,

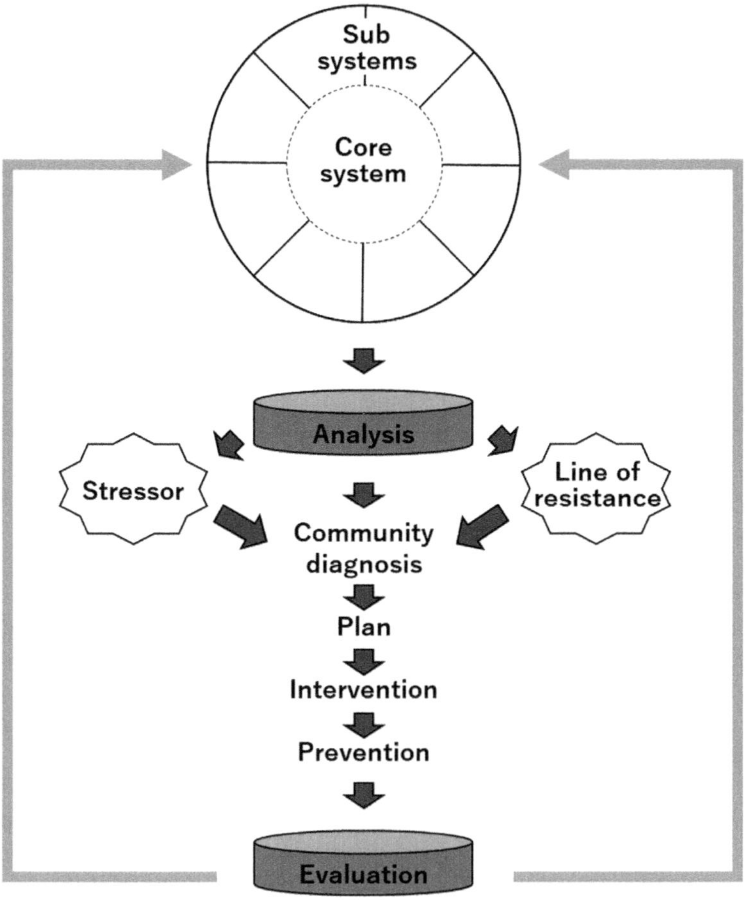

Fig. 2.1 Community as Partner model (Anderson & McFarlane, 2019)

communities can develop solutions that are more attuned to local needs and circumstances. The CAP model not only focuses on addressing immediate health concerns but also aims to empower communities to take charge of their health and well-being in the long term. Through this model, communities develop the skills, knowledge, and confidence to identify their health priorities, advocate for necessary resources, and implement sustainable health initiatives. This empowerment aspect is crucial for building resilient and self-reliant communities.

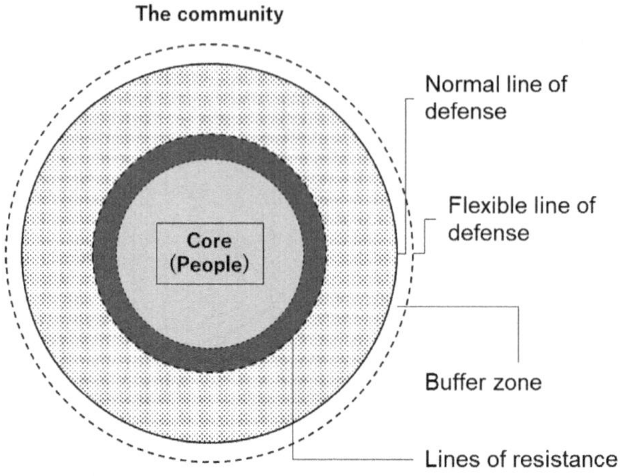

Fig. 2.2 Concept of community and community resilience (Anderson & McFarlane, 2019)

2.6 Human-Centered Design and Community-Based Participatory Research

In public health nursing, it is crucial to understand the social, economic, and environmental factors that underlie the health issues faced by communities. Due to the unique characteristics of each community, a one-size-fits-all approach is inadequate. Instead, customized interventions that align with the local culture, customs, and needs are required. Human-centered nursing research views individuals not merely as isolated entities but as members of a community. This approach aims to assess the health problems they face and the effectiveness of solutions within the context of societal interactions. By focusing on human dignity and individual needs, this method can lead to more effective and sustainable health improvement strategies. This community-based research encourages active participation from residents, reflecting their voices in designing more appropriate and acceptable health promotion programs and interventions. Additionally, respecting the cultural background and values of the community can make health initiatives more meaningful and effective. Human-centered design (HCD) and community-based participatory research (CBPR) (Israel et al., 1998) are two people-centered approaches to addressing real-world problems (Chen et al., 2020). Traditionally, HCD has been used in the private sector, whereas CBPR has been used more commonly by academic and community organizations, often in partnership. HCD (i.e., design thinking) is a repeatable, creative approach to problem-solving that brings together what is desirable from a human point of view with what is technologically feasible and economically viable. CBPR in the health field is a collaborative approach to research that equitably involves all partners in the research process. Both approaches rely on close collaboration between the design team or research team and the beneficiaries and include the deliberate use of cocreation practices, whereby the team and the beneficiaries both contribute directly to the design and development of the outcome or product (Chen et al., 2020).

2.7 Challenges to Inclusiveness Through CBPR

CBPR has the potential to be especially useful in contexts in which cultural diversity and/or socioeconomic disparities are an issue (Washington et al., 2002). This section introduces a past project that challenges LGBTQ inclusiveness using the CBPR approach.

The Unlearning Civic Theatre Project (Haco-Tec) was conducted in Tokyo in 2021 as a collaboration between the theatrical corporation Hakononakanohako and a PHN researcher. Hakononakanohako was a theater management company in Tokyo. Their mission was to learn about society through art products, and their theme in 2021 was about social discrimination against LGBTQ people. In initiating this project, the organizer of this project was concerned about the presence of negative attitudes toward LGBTQ individuals among both company staff and actors. He and the PHN researcher (author) discussed and decided to change the community composed of staff and actors through the theatrical project relevant to LGBTQ actions. These actions were based on the steps of CBPR. The PHN researcher conducted interviews with stakeholders to assess their attitudes and create a list of potential issues. Through discussion with community members (ten members consist of staff and actors), the primary issue to be addressed in their community was developed: the habitual practice of judging individuals based on their LGBTQ identity. The theater program used an existing script that depicted the 25-year journey of a gay man exploring his identity. The PHN researcher engaged in providing feedback to the members to facilitate an easier understanding of the struggles faced by the stakeholders and the societal factors contributing to them (Fig. 2.3). They provided feedback to the members based on qualitative analysis of the script text, past LGBTQ policies, issues in public health, and papers on discrimination against

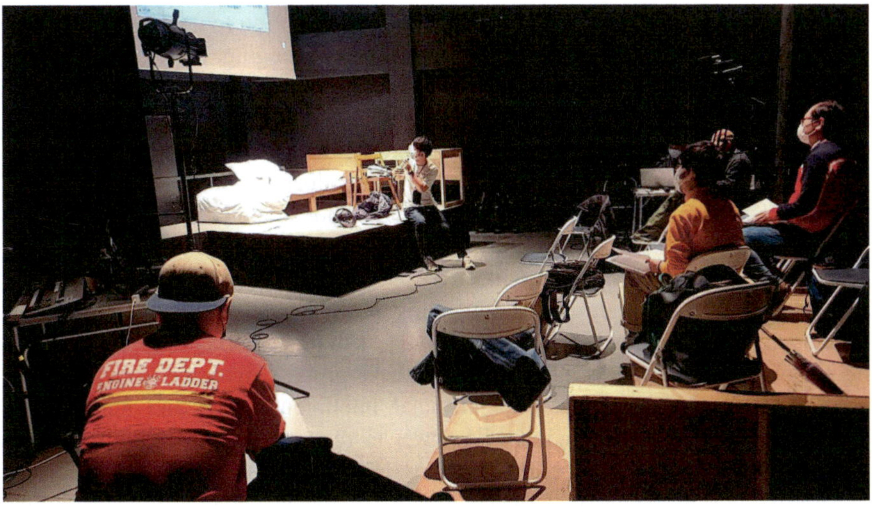

Fig. 2.3 Researcher (center) facilitates group discussion among staff and actors

LGBTQ stakeholders. This led to repeated discussions with the members on directing the play and the significance behind the actors' performances. The project observed changes in staff and actors, such as empathy and modification ("I thought LGBTQ people were from a different world, but realized they are right next to us, in the same community"). The members were motivated to keep challenging social issues, and their activities have continued in community theaters and film.

2.8 Expectations for the Introduction of Digital Technology into Public Health Nursing

In community development adhering to the CBPR approach, it is crucial for researchers and community residents to collaboratively engage in the process of collecting and analyzing community data based on the CAP framework and to make various decisions together. The advent of global digital technologies is anticipated to positively impact this data collection, analysis, and shared decision-making process. The utilization of a Personal Health Record (PHR) (Tang et al., 2006), where individuals manage their own health information, has become an international topic. Previously, individual health information was dispersedly managed by healthcare institutions and individuals. The utilization of PHR involves the development of an environment that is centered around the individual's agreement, focusing on centralized data management and population analysis (Sarwal & Gupta, 2024). Correctly interpreted, PHR has the potential to offer valuable data points for evaluating the clinical trajectory pre-presentation, offering a depth of detail beyond what could be attained solely through conventional patient interviews. This principle stands as an essential aspect of shared decision-making between patients and their healthcare providers (Davis et al., 2017). Similarly, PHR has the potential to contribute to the improvement of CBPR and/or CAP model practice. In past decades, finding the optimal publicly available data when attempting to analyze the current situation in the community diagnosis process was challenging. Particularly for epidemiological data, it is common for only summarized values for specific districts or populations to be published, which sometimes do not provide the information of interest for advancing CAP (General Incorporated Association of PHRC, 2023). In such instances, many CAP projects had to either conduct new surveys themselves or abandon data analysis and decision-making. If various data can be freely utilized within CAP projects in the future, it would significantly enhance the efficiency and accuracy of the community data collection and analysis process. Moreover, having access to appropriate data could potentially improve the quality of community development by strengthening the persuasiveness of new interventions and increasing the number of residents interested in the CAP process. With the advent of technologies, the relationship between artificial intelligence (AI) and humans has become much closer. Leveraging AI's power to review and integrate information posted on the Internet might be advantageous. However, aspects such as the nuances of various emotions people feel, the landscape they live in, and their life aspirations, which are often not digitized, are fundamental to community empowerment. At the heart of community empowerment lies human relationships, where individuals coexist as a community, share with their neighbors, and collectively gain control. The methods to drive this are still to be explored through collaboration between humans and AI.

2.9 Conclusion: The Four Key "Opens" for Human-Centered Public Health Nursing

In response to the diversity of issues inherent in communities, there is a need to establish a system where various stakeholders can transcend their individual perspectives and differences to collaborate effectively. Public health and nursing professionals play a crucial role in this process, working alongside residents to foster communities characterized by inclusiveness and mutual support. As these communities evolve, the distinction between professionals and residents may blur, signaling a shift away from traditional hierarchical structures toward a more collaborative approach.

This evolving landscape necessitates the adoption of "Open Community Development," a paradigm that emphasizes openness and collaboration at every level. This approach is predicated on the understanding that the collective intelligence and capabilities of a community can lead to innovative solutions and sustainable development. Embracing this model requires a commitment to transparency, knowledge-sharing, and inclusivity, ensuring that all voices are heard and valued in the decision-making process.

Open Community Development is underpinned by four key "opens": open governance, open professionalism, open data, and an open mind. Open governance refers to the democratization of decision-making, where community members actively participate in shaping policies and initiatives. Open professionalism involves sharing expert knowledge and skills with the broader community, empowering residents with the information they need to contribute meaningfully. Open data advocates for the free exchange of information, ensuring that community decisions are informed by a comprehensive understanding of local contexts. Lastly, an open mind is the foundational attitude that fosters inclusiveness, empathy, and a willingness to embrace diversity and change. As we move forward, embracing these "opens" will be pivotal in building healthier, more inclusive communities. Open Community Development encourages a culture of collaboration, where diverse perspectives are not only welcomed but are seen as essential to creating holistic and effective solutions. By fostering an environment where everyone feels valued and empowered, we can collectively address the complex challenges facing our communities and pave the way for a more equitable and sustainable future.

Acknowledgments The authors thank Seiko Iimura (research assistant, Kobe City College of Nursing) for her editorial support and literature management. Generative AI tools were used to assist with drafting and language refinement; all content was critically reviewed and approved by the authors. The authors acknowledge colleagues at Sompo Japan and the broader global health community for their insights into resilient health systems.

Author Contributions Conceptualization: Takashi Naruse. Writing—original draft: Takashi Naruse; editorial coordination by Sakiko Kanbara. Writing—review and editing: Sakiko Kanbara; editorial and linguistic assistance provided by a research assistant (Seiko Iimura). Literature search and reference management: research assistant (Seiko Iimura). AI-assisted drafting: Generative AI tools were used to support initial structuring and language refinement under the supervision of the authors.

References

American Public Health Association. (2013). *Public health nursing section. The definition and practice of public health nursing: A statement of the public health nursing section*. American Public Health Association.

American Public Health Association. (2025). *What is public health?* APA. Retrieved April 30, 2025 from https://www.apha.org/what-is-public-health.

Anderson, E. T., & McFarlane, J. (2019). Chapter 11: The process of working with the community. In *Community as partner: Theory and practice in nursing* (8th ed., pp. 173–214). Wolters Kluwer Health.

Braveman, P., Arkin, E., Orleans, T., Proctor, D., & Plough, A. (2017). *What is health equity? And what difference does a definition make?* Princeton.

Bruce, L. (2019). Chapter 6: Community empowerment. In *Community as partner: Theory and practice in nursing* (8th ed., pp. 93–105). Wolters Kluwer Health.

Chen, E., Leos, C., Kowitt, S. D., & Moracco, K. E. (2020). Enhancing community-based participatory research through human-centered design strategies. *Health Promotion Practice., 21*(1), 37–48.

Davis, S., Roudsari, A., Raworth, R., Courtney, K. L., & MacKay, L. (2017). Shared decision-making using personal health record technology: A scoping review at the crossroads. *Journal of the American Medical Informatics Association, 24*(4), 857–866.

Fee, E., & Bu, L. (2010). The origins of public health nursing: The Henry street visiting nurse service. *American Journal of Public Health, 100*(7), 1206–1207.

Gatseva, A. M. (2011). Public health: The science of promoting health. *Journal of Public Health, 19*, 205–206.

General Incorporated Association PHR Council (PHRC). (2023). *Guidelines for PHR service providers* (2nd ed.). General Incorporated Association PHR Council. (in Japanese).

Hassmiller, S. B. (2022). Revitalizing public health nursing for the future. *American Journal of Public Health, 112*(S3), S262–S264.

Institute of Medicine. (1988). *The future of public health*. National Academy Press.

Israel, B. A., Schulz, A. J., Parker, E. A., & Becker, A. B. (1998). Review of community-based research: Assessing partnership approaches to improve public health. *Annual Review of Public Health, 19*, 173–202.

Kulbok, P. A., Thatcher, E., Park, E., & Meszaros, P. (2012). Evolving public health nursing roles: Focus on community participatory health promotion and prevention. *Online Journal of Issues in Nursing, 17*(2), 1.

Laverack, G. (2006). Improving health outcomes through community empowerment: A review of the literature. *Journal of Health, Population, and Nutrition, 24*(1), 113–120.

Ministry of Health, Labour and Welfare. (2023). *The Basic Act on Dementia to Promote an Inclusive Society*. Retrieved April 30, 2025 from https://www.mhlw.go.jp/content/12300000/001119099.pdf (in Japanese).

Ministry of Health, Labour and Welfare. (2025). *Ministry's portal site for Inclusive society*. Retrieved April 30, 2025 from https://www.mhlw.go.jp/kyouseisyakaiportal/#tiikikyosei (in Japanese).
Miyah, Y., Benjelloun, M., Lairini, S., & Lahrichi, A. (2022). COVID-19 impact on public health, environment, human psychology, global Socioeconomy, and education. *The Scientific World Journal, 2022*, 5578284. https://doi.org/10.1155/2022/5578284
National Academies of Sciences, Engineering, and Medicine, National Academy of Medicine. (2021). Committee on the future of nursing. In J. L. Flaubert, S. Le Menestrel, D. R. Williams, & M. K. Wakefeld (Eds.), *The future of nursing 2020–2030: Charting a path to achieve health equity*. National Academies Press (US).
Sarwal, D., & Gupta, V. (2024). Personal health record. In *StatPearls [Internet]*. StatPearls Publishing. Retrieved April 30, 2025 from https://www.ncbi.nlm.nih.gov/books/NBK557757/.
Steward, D. (2022). *Nurses, a voice to lead: Invest in nursing and respect rights to secure global health*. International Council of Nurses.
Tang, P. C., Ash, J. S., Bates, D. W., Overhage, J. M., & Sands, D. Z. (2006). Personal health records: Definitions, benefits, and strategies for overcoming barriers to adoption. *Journal of the American Medical Informatics Association, 13*(2), 121–126.
Washington, A. E., Nápoles-Springer, A., Forté, D. A., Alexander, M., & Pérez-Stable, E. J. (2002). Establishing centers to address treatment effectiveness in diverse ethnic groups: The MEDTEP experience. *Ethnicity & Health, 7*(4), 231–242.
Winslow, C. E. (1920). The untilled fields of public health. *Science, 51*(1306), 23–33.

Open Governance for Human Security: Cultivating JIMOTO Ownership and Surfacing Unconscious Needs in Japan's Local Communities

3

Sakiko Kanbara

3.1 Introduction

In an era defined by unprecedented global connectivity, a paradox has emerged: while risks are increasingly global in origin—climate change, pandemics, financial crises, and technological disruption—their impacts are profoundly local in manifestation. The COVID-19 pandemic exemplified this paradox with stark clarity. A virus that emerged in a single city rippled across the globe within months, yet its effects were experienced most acutely at the neighborhood level: in overwhelmed hospitals, isolated elders unable to receive visits from family, shuttered local businesses that had sustained communities for generations, and food security crises affecting specific marginalized populations.

Similarly, climate change manifests as rising global average temperatures, but its human toll appears in specific localities—flooded villages in Bangladesh and Japan, heatwave-stricken cities in Europe and South Asia, and drought-affected agricultural regions in sub-Saharan Africa and Australia. The 2018 West Japan floods, which we examine in detail later, killed over 200 people and displaced thousands, primarily in Hiroshima, Okayama, and Ehime prefectures. While climate scientists could connect the event to broader patterns of atmospheric warming and increased moisture capacity, the tragedy unfolded house by house, neighborhood by neighborhood—elderly residents trapped in rising waters, evacuation centers struggling with limited supplies, and local nurses working around the clock to provide care amid infrastructure collapse.

This reality has profound implications for disaster nursing and public health. It suggests that strengthening local resilience is not a peripheral concern but a central

S. Kanbara (✉)
Faculty of Nursing, Kobe City College of Nursing, Kobe, Japan
e-mail: s-kanbara@kobe-ccn.ac.jp

S. Kanbara (ed.), *Transformative Community Health Nursing*,
https://doi.org/10.1007/978-3-032-24405-5_3

strategy for managing global risks. As the Sendai Framework for Disaster Risk Reduction (2015–2030) emphasizes:

> Disasters predominantly affect people at the local and community level.... Disaster risk reduction requires that responsibilities be shared by central and local governments, sectors, and stakeholders, as appropriate to their national circumstances and systems of governance. (UNDRR, 2015, Priority 2)

The framework explicitly calls for empowering local authorities and communities, recognizing that effective disaster risk management must be grounded in local knowledge, local capacity, and local ownership. It emphasizes the critical role of "people-centred preventive and multi-hazard approaches" and the need to "strengthen disaster preparedness for response, and to 'Build Back Better' in recovery and reconstruction" (UNDRR, 2015).

Yet in practice, disaster preparedness and health systems often remain centralized, top-down, and disconnected from everyday community life. Plans are written in capital cities by national agencies, assuming uniform conditions and capacities across diverse localities. Community health resources are allocated based on aggregate statistics that mask local variation and marginalized populations. Emergency responses are coordinated through hierarchical command structures that struggle to adapt to messy, context-specific realities on the ground. As one Mabi district resident recounted after the 2018 floods:

> The national disaster plan said to evacuate to the designated shelter. But the shelter was in the affected area. We had to make our own decisions based on what we knew about our neighborhood. (Shaw, 2019)

This disconnect reveals a fundamental flaw in conventional approaches: they treat "local" as a site of policy implementation rather than recognizing it as a source of innovation, resilience, and human security.

3.1.1 Reframing "Local": JIMOTO as Lived Space, Not Administrative Unit

This chapter argues for a fundamental reorientation. We use the Japanese concept of *jimoto* to emphasize that "local" is not merely an administrative scale (municipal, prefectural, or regional) but a lived dimension of everyday life—where routines, relationships, informal care networks, and mutual aid are continuously negotiated.

Jimoto literally means "ground origin" or "local base" (ji = place; moto = origin/source), but its connotations extend far beyond geography. Jimoto evokes:

- Rootedness: the place where one's identity is formed and sustained
- Belonging: feeling "at home," recognized, and embedded in social networks
- Mutual responsibility: caring for and being cared for by neighbors, not as duty but as natural reciprocity
- Local knowledge: understanding the specific conditions, histories, and dynamics of a place in ways that outsiders cannot

To say "this is my *jimoto*" is to claim a relationship of care and commitment to that place and its people. It is not defined by administrative boundaries but by the density of everyday interactions and the sense of shared fate. A *jimoto* might be:

- A neighborhood within a larger city
- A rural village or mountain hamlet
- A school district where parents and teachers know each other's families
- A shopping street where merchants and customers have decades-long relationships
- An online community of residents who coordinate disaster preparedness via social media

What defines *jimoto* is not its size but the quality of lived connection: the informal channels through which information flows, help is sought, and collective action emerges. During the COVID-19 pandemic, for example, many Japanese neighborhoods (particularly in older residential areas) activated *jimoto* networks to check on isolated elders—neighbors leaving notes, shop owners delivering groceries, and community association leaders coordinating phone trees. These actions were not mandated by policy; they emerged from jimoto relationships.

Conversely, the erosion of *jimoto* is often cited as a source of vulnerability in modern Japan. Rapid urbanization, nuclear family structures, long commutes, and digital mediation have weakened face-to-face community ties. In anonymous apartment complexes, residents may not know their neighbors' names. In declining rural areas, the remaining elderly population may lack younger neighbors who could provide support. This thinning of jimoto increases disaster risk: when evacuation orders are issued, who will notice if Mrs. A hasn't left her home? Who will help Mr. B, who uses a wheelchair, navigate evacuation routes? Who will translate emergency information for the Nepali family that moved in last year?

3.1.2 Japan's "Everyday Disasters": Demography as Slow-Moving Crisis

Japan's local communities today face profound challenges that resemble ongoing "everyday disasters"—chronic, slow-moving crises that erode social and economic vitality with the same devastating force as sudden shocks, but over longer timeframes. The most prominent of these is demographic decline.

A landmark 2014 report by the Japan Policy Council, led by former Minister of Internal Affairs and Communications Hiroya Masuda, projected that 896 of Japan's 1727 municipalities—nearly half, concentrated in rural and mountainous areas—could be "at risk of extinction" by 2040 due to severe depopulation among younger generations, particularly women of childbearing age (Masuda, 2014).

The report triggered an intense national debate. While subsequent analyses questioned whether outright "extinction" is predetermined (arguing that migration patterns and birth rates could shift), the warning catalyzed national attention to the crisis of regional decline. In response, the Japanese government launched the local revitalization policy framework in 2014, allocating significant budgets for regional development, population stabilization, and community vitality initiatives.

Yet despite these efforts, demographic pressures persist. Japan's total population peaked at 128 million in 2008 and has been declining since, projected to fall below 100 million by 2053 (National Institute of Population and Social Security Research, 2023). More critically, the distribution is increasingly uneven: Tokyo and surrounding prefectures continue to gain population while most rural prefectures lose people—a pattern that concentrates wealth, services, and opportunities in a shrinking number of urban centers while hollowing out the countryside.

This demographic crisis is not merely a statistical abstraction. It manifests in specific, tangible ways at the community level:

1. *Service Collapse*
   - Schools close as enrollment drops, forcing children to travel long distances or board away from home
   - Public transport routes (buses, local train lines) are discontinued due to lack of ridership, isolating elderly residents without cars
   - Local hospitals and clinics struggle to recruit doctors and nurses; some close entirely, forcing sick residents to travel hours for specialist care
   - Post offices, banks, and shops shut, eroding local economic infrastructure
2. *Infrastructure Decay*
   - Roads, bridges, and water/sewage systems deteriorate as municipal tax revenues decline
   - Abandoned houses proliferate—over 8.5 million nationally in 2018, creating safety and aesthetic blight
   - Agricultural land is abandoned as farming families age out without successors
3. *Cultural Erosion*
   - Traditional festivals scaled back or discontinued as the generation that organized them passes away
   - Craft practices, dialects, and oral histories fade without transmission to younger generations
   - Community institutions (*kōminkan* community centers, volunteer fire brigades) struggle to recruit participants
4. *Care Crisis*
   - Elderly residents living alone become invisible—their isolation is noticed only when mail piles up or a neighbor detects an unusual smell (the phenomenon of lonely death)
   - Family caregivers (often women in their 60s caring for parents in their 80s–90s) face extreme burdens with limited formal support
   - People with disabilities find accessible services scarce as providers consolidate in urban areas
   - Dementia prevalence rises with little infrastructure to support community-based care
5. *Compound Vulnerability*
   - All of the above challenges interact and amplify each other, creating vicious cycles of decline

Critically, these challenges disproportionately affect the most vulnerable. Non-Japanese residents (particularly those with limited Japanese language ability) face compounded exclusion as community networks thin and services centralize. Women bear increased unpaid caregiving burdens. Children in depopulated areas have fewer educational and recreational opportunities. People with chronic illnesses or disabilities lose access to specialized care.

3.1.3 Human Security and the Case for Local Revitalization

What makes these "everyday disasters" particularly syndemic is their gradualism. Unlike earthquakes or floods, which galvanize immediate response and unlock emergency resources, slow-moving crises allow communities to normalize decline. People adjust expectations downward, accepting reduced services and opportunities as inevitable. Out-migration becomes a self-fulfilling prophecy: young people leave because there are no jobs, which leads to business closures, which drives more departures. This creates a vicious cycle where communities lose not only population but also collective agency—the belief that change is possible and that local action matters.

From a human security perspective, this situation is unacceptable. Human security, as defined by the UN Development Programme (UNDP, 1994), shifts the focus from state security (protecting borders and territory) to the security of individuals—ensuring people can live with dignity, free from fear and want. It recognizes that threats to security include not only violence and conflict but also "chronic threats such as hunger, disease, and repression" (UNDP, 1994, p. 23).

The UNDP framework identifies seven dimensions of human security:

1. Economic security: assured basic income and employment
2. Food security: physical and economic access to food
3. Health security: access to health care and protection from disease
4. Environmental security: protection from environmental degradation
5. Personal security: protection from physical violence
6. Community security: protection from ethnic violence and preservation of cultural identity
7. Political security: protection of basic human rights and freedoms

Viewed through this lens, Japan's demographic decline represents a fundamental human security challenge: it systematically erodes people's access to the essential conditions for a dignified life across multiple dimensions—economic (job loss, business closure), food (limited access to fresh groceries in food deserts), health (hospital/clinic closures), environmental (infrastructure decay), community (cultural erosion), and political (reduced civic capacity and representation).

Yet this framing also reveals opportunity. If demographic decline is a form of disaster, then disaster risk reduction principles can be applied:

- *Prevention/Mitigation*: policies to slow depopulation (family support, job creation, and improved quality of life)
- *Preparedness*: building community capacity to adapt to demographic change
- *Response*: targeted interventions during acute crises (e.g., hospital closures)
- *Recovery/Reconstruction*: regenerative approaches that don't just restore pre-crisis conditions but "build back better"

If human security is threatened, then human security strategies become relevant:

- *Participatory governance*: ensuring that affected populations have a voice and agency
- *Protection of rights*: safeguarding access to essential services and cultural dignity
- *Empowerment*: building community capacity for self-determination and collective action

The question becomes: How can communities facing "everyday disasters" cultivate the ownership and capacity needed to not merely survive decline but to regenerate?

3.1.4 JIMOTO Ownership: From Passive Recipients to Active Co-Creators

The concept of jimoto ownership offers a pathway toward this transformation. In the context of local revitalization, strengthening *jimoto* means more than attracting residents or economic investment. It means cultivating a mindset shift from perceiving community problems as external impositions ("someone else's responsibility") to treating them as shared challenges ("our work together").

This ownership is not abstract. It manifests in concrete behaviors:

- Residents attend town meetings not because they are required but because they feel their input matters and could shape outcomes
- Neighbors check on each other not out of formal duty but from genuine concern and reciprocity
- Community members volunteer time to maintain public spaces, organize events, or support vulnerable neighbors because they see their own well-being as inseparable from the well-being of their *jimoto*
- Young people choose to return to or remain in their hometown not despite its challenges but because they see opportunities to make a meaningful difference
- Local businesses invest in community initiatives (sponsoring festivals, supporting schools) because they recognize long-term interdependence with community vitality

Importantly, *jimoto* ownership does not arise from slogans or top-down campaigns. It is built through repeated experiences of meaningful participation—small but tangible instances where people's voices genuinely shape decisions and where collaborative actions produce visible improvements in everyday life:

Example: Disaster Drills
When residents participate in disaster drills that feel relevant to their actual risks and capacities (not generic checklists from national agencies), where they practice helping specific vulnerable neighbors and using local knowledge of evacuation routes, ownership strengthens. They gain confidence: "We know what to do. We can protect each other."

Conversely, *jimoto* ownership erodes when:

- Participation is performative (meetings where decisions are pre-made, "public comment" that is ignored)
- Initiatives fail due to lack of resources or follow-through (volunteers burn out, and promised support does not materialize)
- External actors (governments, corporations, and NGOs) treat communities as passive beneficiaries rather than co-creators
- Success stories are not shared or celebrated, making invisible the positive impact of collective action

3.1.5 Implications for Disaster Nursing and Community Health Practice

This understanding of *jimoto* ownership has direct implications for disaster nursing and community health practice. It suggests that interventions designed to "build community resilience" will fail if they treat communities as passive recipients of expert knowledge and external resources.

Traditional approaches often follow a deficit model:

1. Experts (nurses, public health officials, and disaster managers) identify community needs through external assessments
2. Experts design interventions based on best practices from elsewhere
3. Experts deliver programs to the community ("we will train you in disaster preparedness")
4. Experts evaluate outcomes using pre-determined metrics

When the project ends, external resources withdraw, and community capacity often collapses.

In contrast, a *jimoto* ownership model emphasizes co-creation:

1. Communities and professionals jointly identify needs, drawing on lived experience and local knowledge as well as technical expertise
2. Communities and professionals co-design interventions, adapting "best practices" to local context and priorities

3. Communities lead implementation with professional support (not the reverse)
4. Communities and professionals collaboratively monitor and evaluate, using both quantitative indicators and narrative feedback

When external project funding ends, community capacity and ownership remain because the community built it themselves.

True resilience requires agency: the collective capacity and confidence to identify problems, imagine solutions, mobilize resources, and adapt strategies based on feedback. Nurses and public health professionals, therefore, must shift from a provider-centered model ("we will deliver services to you") to a partnership model ("we will work with you to co-create solutions").

This is where open governance enters the picture. Open governance—characterized by transparency, participation, and collaboration—provides the structural mechanism for cultivating *jimoto* ownership at scale. It creates:

- *Institutional spaces*: Regional Agoras where diverse stakeholders convene as equals
- *Participatory processes*: Design thinking workshops, citizen dialogues, and co-creation methodologies
- *Accountability loops*: Transparent decision-making, public reporting, and continuous feedback mechanisms

The following sections unpack how open governance works in practice and how nursing can contribute to its success.

3.2 Unconscious Needs and the Limits of Conventional Planning

3.2.1 The Problem of "Supply Logic" Versus "Life Logic"

Community planning—whether for health services, disaster preparedness, or social welfare—often begins with what can be easily measured: service utilization rates, disease prevalence, disaster damage assessments, and economic indicators. These metrics are valuable, but they represent supply logic: what governments and organizations can provide, track, and evaluate.

What is frequently missing is life logic: what people actually need to live with dignity, safety, and well-being in their everyday contexts. Life logic includes:

- The informal networks people rely on for childcare, elder care, and emotional support
- The cultural practices that provide meaning and social cohesion
- The subtle barriers (stigma, distrust, language, and literacy) that prevent people from accessing services even when they exist

- The trade-offs people make to survive (skipping meals to pay rent, foregoing medical care due to cost/shame, and hiding vulnerabilities to avoid judgment)
- The latent risks that only become visible during crises (who has no emergency contacts, who cannot evacuate independently, and who will fall through cracks in disaster response)

When planning is dominated by supply logic, the result is a familiar gap: programs exist on paper, while residents feel they do not fit real life. For example:

- A disaster shelter is designated in a school gymnasium, but it is on the far side of a river that floods frequently. Residents with mobility limitations cannot reach it safely.
- Mental health services are available, but only during business hours (impossible for shift workers) and only in Japanese (excluding non-native speakers), and carrying significant stigma (deterring those who fear judgment).
- Nutrition programs provide information about healthy eating but do not address food deserts where fresh produce is unavailable or unaffordable.
- Pandemic infection control guidelines assume private bedrooms and home internet access—luxuries many low-income families lack.

These mismatches are not primarily implementation failures. They are human security risks rooted in the invisibility of unconscious needs.

3.2.2 Defining "Unconscious Needs"

We use the term unconscious needs to refer to needs that are:

1. *Not fully recognized* by the individuals themselves (normalized risks, habits, or conditions that seem inevitable)
2. *Not articulated* in formal planning processes (due to lack of language, lack of confidence, or social/cultural barriers)
3. *Not addressed* by existing services (because they fall outside conventional categories or because services are not reaching those in need)

Unconscious needs overlap with but are distinct from related concepts:

- *Latent needs (*existing but not yet activated): unconscious needs are a subset
- *Unmet needs* (needs that exist but are not addressed): unconscious needs are unmet *because they are not visible*
- *Hidden vulnerabilities* (risks that only become apparent during crises): often rooted in unconscious needs

Why "Unconscious"?

We retain this term (despite earlier drafts to use "unmet needs") because it captures a specific dynamic central to design thinking and field inquiry: these needs are hidden even to those experiencing them. This is different from needs that are recognized but unmet due to resource constraints. Unconscious needs require a different methodological approach—not simply asking "what do you need?" (which assumes people can articulate needs) but engaging in empathetic observation, narrative inquiry, and participatory sensemaking to surface what is not yet consciously understood.

This concept draws on:

- *Design thinking*—people cannot directly answer "why?" questions about choices shaped by unconscious drivers
- *Social epidemiology*: "inverse care law"—those with the greatest need often have the least access, partly because needs are not recognized by systems or individuals
- *Disaster sociology*: vulnerability is often invisible until a crisis reveals it (e.g., who has no social network and who cannot evacuate independently)

3.2.3 Examples of Unconscious Needs in Japanese Communities

Unconscious needs take distinct forms depending on the population context. Among immigrant families, structural invisibility is the primary dynamic: many foreign residents in Japan are entitled to health and disaster services but do not access them, not because of deliberate avoidance but because language barriers, distrust of authorities, and unfamiliarity with local systems prevent articulation of need in formats that planning processes recognize (see Chap. 4 for extended case discussion). Similarly, the digital divide creates information asymmetry that only becomes apparent when a nurse or community worker actively investigates how different groups receive emergency alerts and health updates. An estimated 58% of adults aged 70 and over in Japan report rarely or never using digital devices (MIC, 2022), meaning that COVID-19 vaccination campaigns, disaster warnings, and service information delivered primarily online never reached them—a gap residents themselves had normalized and therefore did not report.

Two further categories of unconscious need are deeply shaped by gender and social norms. Informal caregivers—predominantly women—frequently do not identify their own physical and mental health needs, internalizing caregiving as a duty and perceiving requests for support as personal failure. Japan's estimated 6.3 million informal caregivers often experience depression and exhaustion without seeking help, in part because the support systems available (respite care, counseling) are unknown to them. Social isolation among elderly residents represents a parallel dynamic: the need is not loneliness per se, which many acknowledge, but the absence of regular social contact that would detect emergencies. An isolated elder rarely says

"I need daily check-ins"—this need only becomes visible through observation, network mapping, and the kind of community health visiting described in Chap. 7.

What unites these examples is a shared epistemological challenge: conventional needs assessments—surveys, intake forms, and focus groups—consistently fail to surface unconscious needs because they assume that people can articulate what they require. Design thinking offers a different starting point: observe behavior, map social ecologies, and listen for what is not said before asking what is needed.

3.2.4 Why Unconscious Needs Matter for Human Security and Disaster Resilience

From a human security perspective, unconscious needs represent systematic vulnerabilities that undermine people's freedom from fear and want. When needs remain invisible, inequities deepen: those who can navigate systems receive support; those who cannot, do not. Preventable harms accumulate—social isolation leads to solitary death, digital exclusion becomes missed disaster warnings, and caregiver burnout becomes elder abuse or caregiver collapse. And when institutions repeatedly fail to meet actual needs, public trust erodes—a slow-moving damage that compounds across crises.

From a disaster resilience perspective, unconscious needs are the blind spots in preparedness and response. Emergency plans that assume everyone can read Japanese, use a smartphone, evacuate independently, and rely on a social network will fail the populations who cannot. Post-disaster recovery programs that target "damaged homes" will miss households that were already fragile before the disaster. Surfacing unconscious needs is therefore not a supplementary activity to be pursued when resources allow; it is a prerequisite for intervention that is both effective and equitable.

3.3 Methods to Visualize and Integrate Unconscious Needs: Design Thinking + Field Inquiry

3.3.1 The Complementary Roles of Design Thinking and Logical Thinking

Uncovering unconscious needs requires a different methodological approach than traditional needs assessment (surveys, focus groups, and statistical analysis). It requires design thinking: an empathy-centered, iterative methodology that begins with understanding people's lived experiences before jumping to solutions.

Yet design thinking alone is insufficient for sustainable, accountable governance. Communities also need logical thinking: the analytical discipline that organizes evidence, clarifies assumptions, assesses feasibility and risk, and ensures that solutions are implementable, affordable, and aligned with policy frameworks.

Drawing on traditional nursing research methods and design thinking principles, we propose the following protocol for community health nurses and local practitioners:

There are eight steps on how to surface Unconscious Needs:

Step 1—Begin with the End in Mind: Clarify the Decision
Before collecting data, ask: What decision will this inquiry support? (e.g., what program to build, what budget to propose, and what partnership to pursue). This prevents "research for research's sake" and focuses inquiry on actionable questions.

Example "We need to decide whether to invest in a digital health platform or strengthen non-digital outreach to elderly residents. Our inquiry should help us understand how different populations actually access health information and services."

Step 2—Define the Gap: Articulate the Challenge
State the desired future state and the current state; draft a preliminary challenge statement in the form: "How might we [achieve X] for [population Y] given [constraint Z]?"

Example "How might we ensure that all residents, regardless of digital literacy, receive timely disaster warnings and health information?"

Step 3—Map Existing Knowledge: Collect Secondary Data
Gather statistics, local plans, prior surveys, incident reports, and media coverage. Identify what is known and what is unknown. This prevents duplicating existing research and highlights gaps where primary inquiry is needed.

Example Municipal data shows smartphone penetration by age group but does not reveal *how* seniors without smartphones currently receive information (TV? Neighbors? Not at all?). This gap needs primary inquiry.

Step 4—Select Methods Intentionally: Qual + Quant Balance
Decide what to learn via interviews (depth, context, narratives), observation (actual behavior, environmental factors), focus groups (group dynamics, collective sense-making), or quick surveys (breadth, patterns). Combining methods avoids blind spots.

Example Interviews with isolated seniors reveal barriers to information access; observation of community centers shows how information is actually distributed; a brief survey quantifies the prevalence of digital exclusion.

Step 5—Design Roles and Ethics: Prepare the Team
Assign interviewer, observer, note-taker, and analyst roles. Prepare informed consent procedures, confidentiality agreements, and data handling rules. Ensure psychological safety for participants (especially when discussing sensitive topics like mental health, poverty, and abuse).

Example Two-person teams—one nurse conducts the interview while another takes detailed notes and observes non-verbal cues. Both receive training in trauma-informed interviewing.

Step 6—Conduct Interviews with Depth: Build Rapport and Probe
Use techniques to communicate with nursing care

- *Non-verbal observation*: Notice what people wear, how they speak, and environmental cues (photos, books, and adaptations in their home)
- *Create safety*: Warm greeting, clear time expectations, confidentiality assurance, and "no right/wrong answers" framing
- *Active listening*: Affirmative nods, echoing, empathetic responses ("that must have been difficult"), and open-ended follow-ups
- *Deep probing*: Instead of asking "why?" (which triggers rationalization), ask "what happened?," "how did you feel?," "what did you do next?," and "can you tell me more about that?"
- *Detect incongruence*: If verbal and non-verbal signals don't match (e.g., saying "I'm fine" while looking distressed), gently probe: "You mentioned you're fine, but you seem worried—can you help me understand?"

Step 7—Synthesize and Make Visible: Code and Map
Use qualitative coding to identify patterns in narratives. Create journey maps (documenting a day/week in someone's life), empathy maps (what they say/think/do/feel), or personas (archetypes representing different user groups). Translate findings into user stories ("As a [type of person], I need [something] so that [benefit]") and "How might we...?" questions.

Example From multiple interviews, a pattern emerges: isolated seniors receive health information primarily from TV news (unreliable, fragmented) or not at all. User story: "As an 80-year-old living alone without internet, I need a trusted person to regularly update me on local health services and disaster preparedness so that I don't miss critical information." HMW question: "How might we create a neighborhood-based information network that doesn't rely on digital access?"

Step 8—Return Results to the Community: Validate and Refine
Before moving to solution design, share findings with community members (in accessible formats—visual posters, short videos, oral presentations, and plain language summaries). Ask: "Does this reflect your experience? What did we miss? What matters most?" This builds trust, corrects blind spots, and ensures that problem definition is co-created, not imposed.

Example Present findings at a Regional Agora session, showing journey maps and direct quotes (anonymized). Invite participants to add sticky notes with corrections, additions, or priorities. Use this feedback to refine the challenge statement before proceeding to ideation.

3.4 Integrated People-Centered Health Services as the Policy Bridge

3.4.1 From Fragmented Systems to Integrated, Accountable Care

Chapter 1 introduced WHO's Integrated People-Centered Health Services (IPCHS) framework as a global strategy to shift health systems toward integrated, life-course care (WHO, 2016). Chapter 2 demonstrated how community-centered nursing practice operationalizes this shift. Chapter 3 now identifies the critical enabling condition: governance arrangements that allow communities to co-decide priorities, coordinate across sectors, and continuously learn. Among IPCHS's five strategic directions, Direction 2—strengthening governance and accountability—is where open governance becomes operationally essential. Without it, person-centered care remains fragile, dependent on individual champions or short-term project funding rather than embedded in sustainable institutional practice.

3.4.2 IPCHS in Disaster and Emergency Contexts

In disaster and emergency contexts, the value of IPCHS is best understood through the lens of the WHO Health Emergency and Disaster Risk Management (HEDRM) framework, which stipulates health systems strengthening—not just emergency response—as the foundation of disaster resilience (WHO, 2019). Traditional disaster response operates through vertical command structures, sector silos, and supply-push models that deliver pre-packaged relief based on generalized assumptions about community needs. These approaches struggle with local adaptation and frequently miss the most vulnerable. HEDRM, by contrast, calls for horizontal coordination across sectors, community participation in needs assessment and service design, and the integration of disaster preparedness into routine health systems—not as a bolt-on "emergency plan" but as a feature of how primary health care, long-term care, and social services are designed and governed day to day.

This integration is operationally important because, as the Sendai Framework emphasizes, "disaster risk reduction practices need to be multi-hazard and multisectoral, inclusive and accessible" (UNDRR, 2015, Priority 4). For nursing and health policy, it means that routine services must be disaster-resilient—able to continue with minimal disruption—while disaster preparedness must build the human capacity, governance structures, and community trust that allow "Build Back Better" recovery to reduce pre-existing vulnerabilities rather than merely restore them.

3.4.3 Open Governance as IPCHS Direction 2 in Action

Building on Okumura's concept of open governance as "practical democracy," this section introduces the Regional Agora as a repeatable design for civic participation (Okumura, 2024). Open governance through Regional Agoras operationalizes IPCHS Direction 2 by creating the concrete mechanisms that transform stated principles into sustained practice: transparent participation across diverse stakeholders, cross-sector coordination that prevents siloed problem-solving, shared accountability through public documentation and community monitoring, and continuous learning through community-reported feedback and iterative adjustment. Table 3.1 shows how design thinking and logical thinking work together across these IPCHS implementation phases—design thinking to surface what genuinely matters to people, and logical thinking to ensure that responses are feasible, accountable, and scalable. This integration is especially critical in nursing, where professionals must navigate between care ethics and public health ethics, clinical judgment and evidence-based protocol, and empathy and professional boundaries. Regional Agoras provide the governance infrastructure to make this navigation a collective, institutionalized practice rather than an individual burden.

Table 3.1 Integrating design thinking and logical thinking in nurse-led open governance for IPCHS

Phase	Design thinking (human desirability)	Logical thinking (feasibility and accountability)	Typical outputs
1. Frame the challenge	Empathy goals: Who matters? What feels unsafe/unfair?	Define scope, constraints, decision points, data sources	Challenge statement; stakeholder map; preliminary indicators
2. Discover needs	Interviews, observation, narratives, journey mapping	Baseline indicators, gap analysis, risk assessment, policy review	Needs map; user personas; evidence brief; literature review
3. Ideate solutions	Divergent brainstorming, wild options, co-creation workshops	Assumption testing, cost/risk screening, alignment with policy frameworks	Option set; selection criteria; feasibility matrix
4. Prototype and pilot	Low-fidelity prototypes, role-play scenarios, service blueprints	Implementation logic, resource plan, privacy/ethics check	Prototype package; pilot protocol; consent forms
5. Test and evaluate	User feedback sessions, story-based evaluation, experience narratives	Indicator tracking, cost-effectiveness analysis, compliance monitoring	Evaluation report; user testimonials; performance data
6. Institutionalize and scale	Embed co-creation as routine civic practice, celebrate success	Governance rules, sustainable budgets, transparency mechanisms, training	Policy adoption; sustained programs; regenerative capacity; public dashboard

This dual approach is especially critical in nursing, where professionals must navigate between care ethics and public health ethics, clinical judgment and evidence-based practice, and empathy and boundaries. Nurses skilled in both can lead transformative change.

IPCHS provides the policy framework for integrating person- and community-centered care. By integrating design thinking and logical thinking across implementation phases, communities can discover what people truly need (human desirability) while ensuring solutions are feasible, sustainable, and accountable (institutional viability).

The next section explores the practical structure of Regional Agoras: how they function as spaces for practical democracy and what principles guide their operation.

3.5 Diversity Management as Governance Capacity

Professor Hirokazu Okumura conceptualizes open governance as "practical democracy" (jissen minshushugi): democracy not as an abstract ideal realized only through periodic elections but as daily practice of shared problem-solving where citizens and officials work side by side as equals (Okumura, 2026). Many citizens experience democracy as distant—voting every few years but having little voice in everyday decisions affecting their lives. Practical democracy seeks to reverse this by creating concrete experiences where participation produces visible results. The Regional Agora—a civic forum where diverse stakeholders engage in collaborative governance—embodies this vision.

Open governance requires more than transparency—it demands practical capacity to manage diversity in participation. Simply creating "spaces for participation" often reproduces existing inequalities, a participation paradox where those with time, education, social capital, and digital access dominate, while marginalized groups (working poor, immigrants, caregivers, digitally excluded elderly, and people with disabilities) remain absent or silent due to structural barriers. The result is elite capture: participatory governance dominated by the already-privileged, inadvertently harming those not at the table.

Diversity management is therefore a core governance capacity—the deliberate, ongoing design work to ensure differences in language, culture, disability, age, gender, and digital literacy do not become exclusion mechanisms. It requires active design across five dimensions:

1. Diversity of Participation (Who is at the table?): Stakeholder mapping, targeted recruitment, schedule flexibility, childcare/transportation support, compensation, and accessible venues
2. Diversity of Information (Accessibility): Simple language, multilingual materials, multiple formats (visual, audio, print, video), interpretation services, and accessible data dashboards

3. Diversity of Decision-Making (Who sets the agenda?): Open agenda-setting, community-led issue identification, rotating priorities, and veto power over external agendas
4. Safety and Silence Management (Psychological safety): Co-created ground rules, active facilitation (round-robin, small groups, anonymous input), conflict management, and validating vulnerability
5. Equity in Data Utilization (Democratizing data literacy): Data transparency, community workshops, resident-led data collection, data storytelling, and welcoming challenges to expert analyses

Without such governance capacity, co-creation remains limited to those with existing privilege—reproducing inequity under the name of participation.

Why this matters for unconscious needs: Diversity management is epistemologically essential for surfacing hidden vulnerabilities. Unconscious needs are often held by precisely those absent from planning—isolated elderly, immigrants with language barriers, informal caregivers, and people with stigmatized conditions. Homogeneous groups have collective blind spots; they cannot surface what they don't experience. If Regional Agoras replicate existing power structures, they replicate existing solutions—which have already failed to address unconscious needs.

This governance-level diversity management connects to Chap. 4's focus on cultural competency at the practice level: how individual providers build trust and deliver culturally appropriate care. System design (Chap. 3) and cultural communication skills (Chap. 4) are both necessary.

For practical implementation guidance, see Box 3.1 (7-step Agora-to-implementation cycle) and Box 3.2 (COG-style proposal template), which provide step-by-step protocols for converting community dialogue into actionable programs (Okumura, 2024).

Box 3.1: The Agora-to-Implementation Method—A 7-Step Cycle for Nurse-Led Social Innovation

This cycle connects the Regional Agora dialogue to concrete action, ensuring that participation produces tangible results rather than remaining discussion-only.

Step 0—Convene: Build the Coalition

Form a minimal cross-sector team including residents, nurses, municipality representatives, and academic or industry partners. Start small (5–10 committed individuals) and grow organically.

Step 1—Sense: Surface Unconscious Needs

Use COG-style template (Box 3.2) to collect lived narratives, conduct observations, and gather open data. Focus on "everyday disasters" and quiet vulnerabilities that formal statistics miss.

(continued)

Box 3.1 (continued)

Step 2—Define: Agree on the Challenge

Through Agora sessions, synthesize findings into a single, testable challenge statement with clear success criteria (equity, dignity, and feasibility). Use "How might we...?" framing to invite creative solutions.

Step 3—Co-Design: Generate and Select Options

Facilitate divergent ideation (brainstorm many possibilities without immediate judgment), then converge on one or two prototypes using transparent selection criteria (impact, cost, feasibility, and equity).

Step 4—Prototype: Build Low-Cost Pilots

Create minimal viable versions—service blueprints, digital mockups, workflow diagrams, and governance rules. Test internally before public launch.

Step 5—Pilot: Run the Intervention

Implement in a limited scope (one neighborhood, 1 month, and a small user group) with diversity management built in (ensure online/offline access, multilingual support, and accessibility).

Step 6—Decide and Scale: Evaluate and Iterate

Collect quantitative outcomes (participation rates, service utilization, and health indicators) and qualitative feedback (stories, satisfaction, and unexpected effects). Report results transparently to the Agora. Decide collectively: scale up, revise and retry, or stop.

Step 7 (Implicit Loop): Return to Step 1

Continuous improvement—what new needs emerged during the pilot? What unexpected barriers appeared?

Key Success Factor: Embed nurses as rotating stewards who facilitate each step, ensuring clinical expertise, care ethics, and community trust are maintained throughout.

Box 3.2: Converting Community Dialogue into Fundable Proposals—COG-Style Templates Adapted for Nursing

The Challenge Open Governance (COG) format forces teams to connect ideas to evidence and implementation plans (COG, 2022). Here is how nurses can adapt it:

WHAT—Service/Activity Description (Public-Facing)

Describe concretely what will happen: Who does what, for whom, where, when, and how? Write a scenario:

(continued)

Box 3.2 (continued)

Every Saturday morning, a community health nurse and trained volunteers will staff a 'health room' in the Tanaka neighborhood community center. Residents can drop in for blood pressure checks, health consultations, and information about local services. Multilingual materials and interpretation will be available.

WHY—Evidence and Rationale (Data + Stories)

Combine quantitative indicators (demographics, service gaps, health statistics) with qualitative evidence (interview quotes, photos, journey maps). State sources clearly.

Municipal data shows 35% of Tanaka ward residents are over 65, with the highest rates of hypertension in the city. Yet the nearest clinic is 3 km away with no direct bus route. Our interviews revealed that 12 of 15 elderly residents interviewed had not seen a doctor in over a year due to transportation barriers and cost concerns. One resident stated: 'I know my blood pressure is high, but I don't want to burden my daughter to drive me to the city clinic.'

HOW—Implementation Pathway (Actors, Resources, Timeline)

- *Who Leads*: *Community Health Nurse Sato* (coordinator), supported by *six trained volunteers*
- *Resources Needed*: Community center space, blood pressure monitors, multilingual pamphlets, and volunteer training
- *Timeline*: Months 1–2 (recruit and train volunteers), Month 3 (soft launch), and Months 4–12 (full operation and evaluation)
- *Partners*: Municipal Health Department (supervision), Tanaka Neighborhood Association (outreach), and Local Pharmacy (donated supplies)

Nursing-Specific Add-Ons

1. *Care Ethics and Safety*: How will the program protect dignity, privacy, and psychosocial well-being? (E.g., *consultations in private rooms, strict confidentiality protocols, referrals to social services for those revealing hardship*)
2. *Diversity Management*: How will participation and services remain accessible across language, disability, and digital divides? (E.g., *non-Japanese speakers paired with bilingual volunteers, wheelchair-accessible venue, both in-person and phone consultation options*)
3. *Learning System*: What indicators will be tracked? How will results be shared? How will governance adapt? (E.g., *monthly attendance, blood pressure control rates, user satisfaction surveys; quarterly public reports to Agora; biannual program review with community input*)

3.6 Conclusion: Open Governance as the Next Frontier in Transformative

This chapter has argued that open governance is the structural mechanism through which person-centered care becomes sustainable community transformation. We began by reframing "local" not as an administrative scale but as jimoto—a lived dimension of everyday relationships and mutual aid—and positioned Japan's demographic decline as a slow-moving human security crisis that calls for the same analytical seriousness as acute disasters. We introduced unconscious needs as the hidden vulnerabilities that conventional planning systematically misses and offered an eight-step protocol for surfacing them through design thinking and field inquiry. We connected WHO's IPCHS framework to Regional Agoras as governance infrastructure and argued that diversity management—active, designed, and continuous—is the condition under which open governance can actually function rather than merely appear to function.

For the nursing profession, this implies a broadened professional identity: from providers within systems to conveners and designers of systems themselves. Nurses hold community trust, bridge clinical and social domains, practice care ethics daily, and navigate complexity routinely—all capacities directly transferable to open governance facilitation. The chapters that follow show what this looks like in practice: in multicultural community care (Chap. 4), digital inclusion in rural settings (Chap. 5), gender-responsive disaster planning (Chap. 6), and citizen-led data initiatives in post-disaster recovery (Chap. 7). Open governance is not a governance theory added on top of nursing—it is the next frontier of what nursing has always done.

Acknowledgments The authors gratefully acknowledge Prof. Hirokazu Okumura for his foundational philosophy of Open Governance and Challenge Open Governance (COG), as well as for his generous guidance and intellectual inspiration throughout the development of this chapter, and his ongoing work in developing practical tools for civic participation and community resilience.

The author thanks Seiko Iimura (research assistant, Kobe City College of Nursing) for her essential support in literature coordination, reference management, and manuscript preparation. Generative AI tools assisted with drafting and language refinement; all content was critically reviewed, revised, and approved by the author. The author also thanks community partners across Japan whose experiences of local governance and mutual aid inspired the concepts developed in this chapter.

Author Contributions Conceptualization: Sakiko Kanbara. Writing—original draft: Sakiko Kanbara. Writing—review and editing: Sakiko Kanbara; editorial and linguistic assistance provided by a research assistant (Seiko Iimura). Literature search, reference management, and manuscript preparation: research assistant (Seiko Iimura). AI-assisted drafting: Generative AI tools were used to support structuring and language refinement under the supervision of Sakiko Kanbara.

Glossary of Japanese Terms

Romanization	English translation	Context/notes
chiho-sosei	Local revitalization	National policy framework launched in 2014 to address regional depopulation
chiiki agora	Regional Agora	Okumura's civic forum model for open governance
honne	True feelings/opinions	As opposed to *tatemae* (official positions), what one privately believes
jimoto	Local place; hometown	Connotes place-based identity, belonging, rootedness
jissen demorakushii	Practical democracy	Okumura's concept: democracy as daily practice, not just elections
kaso	Depopulation; underpopulation	Describes rural areas experiencing severe population decline
kodokushi	Lonely death; solitary death	Phenomenon of elderly people dying alone, undiscovered for extended periods
kojo	Public aid/assistance	Government-provided disaster support (part of jijo-kyojo-kojo framework)
kyojo	Mutual aid	Community-level disaster support (neighbors helping neighbors)
jijo	Self-help	Individual/household-level disaster preparedness
shōmetsu kanou toshi	Cities at risk of extinction	Term from the Masuda Report for municipalities facing severe depopulation
tatemae	Official position; public facade	As opposed to *honne*; what one expresses publicly regardless of private belief
tōjisha ishiki	Stakeholder consciousness	Taking ownership; seeing oneself as a responsible actor rather than a passive observer

References

Challenge Open Governance (COG). (2022). *Proposal entry sheet format ("What/Why/How") used for citizen-participatory innovation proposals* (Japanese). https://park.itc.u-tokyo.ac.jp/padit/cog2022/final/idea/46_idea.pdf

Masuda, H. (2014). *Regional cities will disappear by 2040: Regional revitalization as urgent policy issue*. Discuss Japan—Japan Policy Forum.

Ministry of Internal Affairs and Communications, Japan (MIC). (2022). *Communications usage trend survey*. https://www.soumu.go.jp/johotsusintokei/tsusin_riyou/data/eng_tsusin_riyou02_2022.pdf

National Institute of Population and Social Security Research (NIPSSR). (2023). *Population projections for Japan: 2021–2070*. https://www.ipss.go.jp/pp-zenkoku/e/zenkoku_e2023/pp2023e_Summary.pdf

Okumura, H. (2024). *Challenge Open Governance: Regional Agora and practical democracy* (Japanese). https://drive.google.com/drive/folders/1qvgr1zivyxm1mnw9qar1ittqcdjmku-8

Okumura, H. (2026). *Open governance as practical democracy: Philosophical foundations of Regional Agora* (Working Paper v7.0). Challenge!! Open Governance.

Shaw, R. (2019). *Interview: Mabi district recovery project reports*. Kurashiki City Government. https://rajibshaw.org/wpRS/wp-content/uploads/2019/02/b60762a38aefaf40ac602aeef2fbf161.pdf

United Nations Development Programme (UNDP). (1994). *Human development report 1994: New dimensions of human security*. Oxford University Press. New York.

United Nations Office for Disaster Risk Reduction (UNDRR). (2015). *Sendai framework for disaster risk reduction 2015–2030*. United Nations.

World Health Organization (WHO). (2016). *Framework on integrated people-centred health services (Document A69/39)*. Report by the Secretariat, Sixty-ninth World Health Assembly.

World Health Organization (WHO). (2019). *Health emergency and disaster risk management framework*. World Health Organization.

Nursing Insights into Community Care in a Globalizing Society

4

Sushila Paudel and Sakiko Kanbara

4.1 Introduction

Japan, known for its vulnerability to natural disasters, has seen a steady increase in its foreign resident population from about 2.0 million in 2012 to nearly 4.0 million by June 2025 (ISA, 2025). This demographic shift presents unique challenges in disaster preparedness and response, particularly in ensuring equitable access to health services and information during crises. The devastating impact of the 2011 Great East Japan Earthquake, the 2018 floods, and the more recent COVID-19 pandemic have highlighted the specific vulnerabilities faced by foreign residents during disasters. Language barriers, lack of local networks, and unfamiliarity with local systems often result in these communities being disproportionately affected. For instance, during the 2011 earthquake, many foreign residents reported difficulties in accessing critical information and emergency services due to language barriers (Shah & Murao, 2013).

Figure 4.1 provides a compact snapshot of Japan's growing foreign resident population and highlights why inclusive community care and disaster risk reduction (DRR) require attention to geographic concentration and diversity in residence status.

Disaster nursing, an evolving field that integrates principles of disaster management with nursing care, plays a crucial role in addressing these challenges. It focuses on providing culturally sensitive care and support to diverse populations before, during, and after disasters. However, the intersection of disaster nursing, PHC, and the specific needs of foreign residents remains an area requiring further exploration and development in Japan. Currently, Japan has initiated several programs aimed at

S. Paudel
Faculty of Nursing, University of Kochi, Kochi, Japan

S. Kanbara (✉)
Faculty of Nursing, Kobe City College of Nursing, Kobe, Japan
e-mail: s-kanbara@kobe-ccn.ac.jp

S. Kanbara (ed.), *Transformative Community Health Nursing*,
https://doi.org/10.1007/978-3-032-24405-5_4

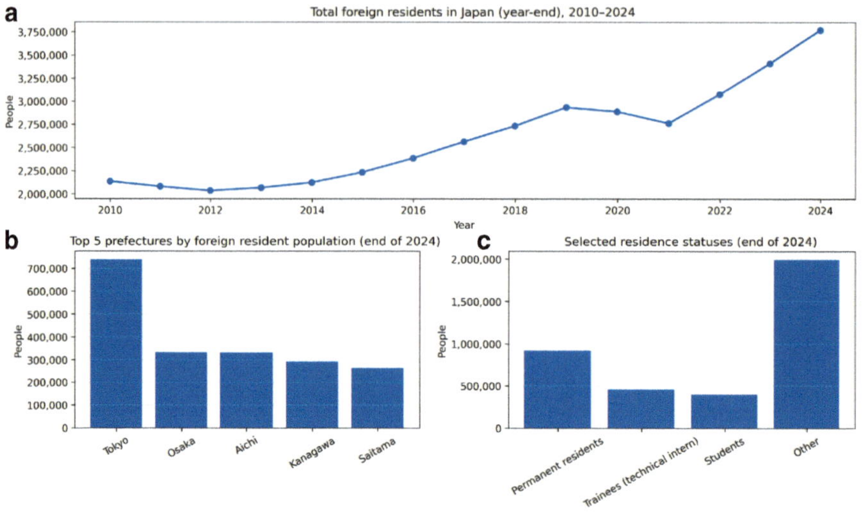

Fig. 4.1 Foreign resident population in Japan: trend, geographic concentration, and residence-status composition. (Source: Immigration Services Agency of Japan (2025). Compiled by authors)

supporting foreign residents during disasters, such as multilingual emergency alert systems (CLAIR, 2024) and disaster preparedness training for international communities. These efforts often lack integration with broader health care systems and community-based approaches.

On top of the existing challenges, the COVID-19 pandemic significantly burdened health services across physical, mental, economic, and social dimensions. This has further emphasized the critical importance of strengthening PHC to maintain the resilience of health systems during crises (OECD, 2021). The World Bank also highlights the necessity of increased investment in PHC (Barış et al., 2022).

4.2 Theoretical Foundations: Cultural Competence and Disaster Nursing in Multicultural Contexts

Nursing in multicultural societies requires theoretical frameworks that recognize both the universal aspects of human dignity and health and the culturally specific meanings of care, illness, and well-being. This section outlines the conceptual foundations that guide nursing practice in diverse communities, particularly during disasters and public health emergencies.

4.2.1 Cultural Competence and Transcultural Nursing

Cultural competence in nursing refers to an ongoing process of developing knowledge, skills, and attitudes that enable respectful, equitable, and effective care for people from diverse backgrounds. It is not a fixed checklist but rather a commitment to continuous learning, self-reflection, and partnership with the communities nurses serve. The International Council of Nurses (ICN) Code of Ethics (2021) grounds this commitment in principles of human rights, non-discrimination, equity, and social justice, calling on nurses to uphold dignity for all individuals and to address systemic inequities in health care access and outcomes.

Leininger's transcultural nursing theory provides a practical framework for culturally congruent care. It emphasizes understanding how different cultural groups perceive health, illness, and care practices, and recognizes that effective nursing requires adapting interventions to align with patients' values, beliefs, and lived experiences. In disaster and Primary Health Care (PHC) contexts, transcultural nursing serves as an operational bridge: it connects routine health promotion and prevention activities with emergency preparedness, response, and recovery. This bridge is essential because communication pathways and care systems that function in everyday situations often break down during crises—particularly for populations facing language barriers, unfamiliar administrative processes, or limited social networks.

The shared foundations of cultural competence and disaster nursing include:

Responding to structural inequities: Recognizing that vulnerabilities during disasters are shaped by pre-existing social, economic, and institutional inequalities, not merely by individual characteristics or nationality.

Partnership with communities: Shifting from a provider-centered model to collaborative relationships where foreign residents and marginalized groups are active participants in planning, decision-making, and safety co-production.

Critical awareness of power relations: Reflecting on how professional authority, language dominance, legal status, and systemic barriers shape access to care and information, and working to reduce these imbalances.

Upholding human dignity and rights: Ensuring that all individuals—regardless of residence status, language proficiency, or cultural background—are treated as rights-holders with inherent worth and agency.

4.3 Disaster Nursing as Culturally Embedded Practice

Disaster nursing extends beyond acute emergency response to encompass long-term, person-centered care that accounts for the social and cultural contexts shaping people's vulnerability and resilience. Disasters affect not only physical health but also social relationships, livelihoods, mental well-being, and cultural identity. Recovery is a prolonged process, often lasting months or years, during which survivors face challenges such as income loss, housing instability, food insecurity, disrupted medication access, and deteriorating mental health (Science Council of Japan, 2013; Ochi et al., 2013).

Foreign residents may face intensified challenges during disasters due to language barriers, unfamiliarity with local systems, limited integration into neighborhood-based mutual aid networks, and precarious legal or employment status. These vulnerabilities are not inherent characteristics but reflect structural conditions—such as exclusion from decision-making processes, inadequate multilingual information channels, and fragmented social support—that can be addressed through inclusive, equity-oriented disaster risk reduction.

Disaster nursing aligns with the concept of human security, which emphasizes protection, empowerment, and dignity across health, social, and economic domains. While clinical care addresses immediate medical needs, the human security perspective highlights the importance of social relationships, community engagement, and long-term well-being. Both approaches are necessary and complementary. The Sendai Framework for Disaster Risk Reduction similarly calls for inclusive, people-centered governance and investment in resilience-building that safeguards lives, health, and living conditions for all populations, including those who may be disproportionately affected (UNDRR, 2015).

In practice, culturally embedded disaster nursing involves identifying and addressing barriers throughout all disaster phases. During preparedness, this includes mapping language diversity, establishing communication channels with trusted community leaders, training health workers in cultural competence, and developing accessible multilingual materials. During a response, it requires providing clear, multilingual information in shelters and clinics, addressing misinformation and stigma, and linking health services with legal or social support when needed. During recovery, culturally responsive care supports continuity for chronic conditions and mental health, follows up on preventive services, and incorporates equity-focused evaluation into PHC systems and local disaster plans. These actions reflect a commitment to disaster nursing not as a temporary intervention but as an integral, sustained dimension of health systems strengthening in multicultural societies.

4.3.1 Cultural Competence in Disaster Settings

Key components of cultural competence in disaster and PHC settings include:

Self-awareness and partnership: Nurses reflect on their own assumptions, power relationships, and biases, approaching care as a collaborative partnership. They are aware of how residence status, regulations, and systemic barriers affect access, connecting people with appropriate support when needed.

Culturally responsive communication and care: Nurses work effectively with interpreters and multilingual resources, using clear language and confirmation techniques. They explore how individuals understand illness and treatment, respect diverse decision-making practices, and negotiate care plans that are both medically sound and culturally acceptable.

Trust-building and crisis-ready inclusivity: Nurses address discrimination and misinformation by partnering with cultural mediators and community leaders.

During emergencies, they adapt triage, shelter support, and continuity-of-care planning to meet diverse needs (diet, medication, mental health, and safety).

For detailed discussions of organizational diversity management and governance frameworks, see Chap. 3. For technology-enabled approaches to reducing information barriers and addressing the digital divide, see Chap. 5.

4.4 Challenges of Access to Health Care and Supportive Relationships in the COVID-19 Pandemic from a Multicultural Nursing Practice Perspective

Building on this cultural and social understanding of disaster nursing, the next section examines concrete barriers to health care access and supportive relationships experienced by foreign residents during the COVID-19 pandemic. Globally, migrants are often considered vulnerable and face inequality, lack of health care, poor economic conditions, discrimination, and violence (Marmot, 2007; Koh, 2020). These challenges are further complicated by individual, structural, and situational factors such as age, gender, literacy, and differences in economic, political, social, and environmental conditions (IOM, 2011). These factors increase the risk of health disadvantages and diseases in the host country. Traditionally, foreign migrants encounter significant barriers to accessing health care, influenced by cultural differences in medical practices and perceptions (Lebano et al., 2020). Access to health care remains a fundamental human right and an essential aspect of health policy and health services research (OHCHR, 2008; WHO, 2017).

Disasters and public health emergencies often amplify pre-existing vulnerabilities. For foreign residents, disruptions in information flows, mobility, income, and access to formal services can quickly translate into delayed care, preventable complications, and avoidable suffering. From a health equity perspective, the goal is not merely to provide the same information or services to everyone but to reduce avoidable gaps that stem from structural and social determinants (Marmot, 2007). Professional nursing ethics reinforce this responsibility. Nurses are expected to provide care without discrimination, protect privacy and dignity, and communicate clearly and responsibly, including through the appropriate use of technology (ICN, 2021). In disaster contexts, these ethical commitments become particularly important, as fear, uncertainty, and misinformation can erode trust and further limit access to care. At the system level, disaster risk reduction frameworks such as the Sendai Framework emphasize integrating risk understanding and governance into health strategies across preparedness, response, and recovery (UNDRR, 2015). To examine these access challenges in a structured way, this chapter applies a four-domain framework that links common barriers faced by foreign residents to corresponding nursing and Primary Health Care (PHC) interventions and measurable indicators (Table 4.1). The framework covers institutional barriers, language and information barriers, issues of culture and trust, and disaster-specific constraints. Cultural competence is treated as a cross-cutting capability that strengthens nursing responses

Table 4.1 Healthcare access barriers for foreign residents: a four-domain framework

Barrier domain (4 domains)	Typical challenges → Nursing/PHC interventions	Example indicators (process/outcome)
Institutional (insurance, eligibility, documentation, pathways)	Challenges: unclear insurance enrollment/coverage; complex procedures and appointment systems; eligibility/documentation gaps; administrative bottlenecks during crises. Interventions: "system navigation" support; insurance/benefit enrollment assistance; clear explanations of entitlements and confidentiality; referral and follow-up pathways; contingency planning for emergencies (medication lists, contacts); flexible policies and outreach during disasters	Process: % enrolled in insurance; % receiving navigation support; time from symptom onset to first consultation. Outcome: avoidable emergency visits; delayed-care reports; patient-reported access experience
Language and information (interpretation, risk communication, digital access)	Challenges: limited Japanese proficiency; variable availability/quality of interpretation; unreadable translations; infodemic and misinformation; digital divide. Interventions: trained interpreters and clear access pathways; multilingual materials and "easy Japanese"; pictograms; two-way communication (hotlines, chat); community information brokers and peer supporters; multilingual alerts through trusted channels	Process: interpreter coverage (hours/availability); % key materials available in multiple languages/easy Japanese; reach of alerts by language. Outcome: comprehension checks; adherence to public health measures; reduced misinformation-related anxiety
Culture and trust (health beliefs, help-seeking, stigma, relationships)	Challenges: different health beliefs/medical system expectations; fear of discrimination; privacy concerns; stigma (including around mental health or infectious disease). Interventions: culturally congruent education; shared decision-making; use of cultural mediators; staff training in cultural competence and trauma-informed communication; respectful inquiry about beliefs and preferences	Process: staff training completion; use of cultural mediators; screening for concerns. Outcome: satisfaction/trust; uptake of preventive services; continuity of care
Disaster-specific constraints (shelters, displacement, continuity of care)	Challenges: sudden loss of routines and resources; disruption of medication supply and chronic care; limited culturally appropriate spaces/food; transport and mobility barriers; exclusion from informal networks. Interventions: multilingual shelter triage and briefings; liaison roles for foreign residents; continuity-of-care support (medicine, referrals); mobile clinics and outreach; inclusive shelter management and protection pathways	Process: time to triage; % shelters with multilingual briefing; continuity-of-care documentation rate. Outcome: preventable complications; mental distress; equitable access to relief and follow-up care

across all four domains by supporting equitable access, continuity of care, and trust-building during crises.

The Japanese healthcare system is known for its high standards and universal coverage. However, its accessibility is primarily for native speakers, inadvertently excluding those unfamiliar with Japanese healthcare practices and language. Language barriers, in particular, hinder effective communication, making it harder for non-native speakers to understand medical practices and accurately communicate symptoms. The pandemic highlighted the need for healthcare providers to improve their cultural competence and to advocate for addressing the social determinants that affect the health of migrants. This includes working with local health care providers, community health centers, and NGOs to enhance service delivery to diverse populations. However, challenges such as illiteracy, inequality, racism, xenophobia, and privacy concerns complicate these efforts (Blomberg et al., 2021; Guadagno, 2020; Bahar et al., 2020; Germain & Yong, 2020). During the COVID-19 pandemic, the need for isolation to prevent transmission created unique difficulties in transmitting information and accessing medical care. Migrants with limited language skills often relied on inadequate or informal sources of information, exacerbating disparities and limiting their ability to seek appropriate care. This situation was further complicated by the spread of misinformation about the virus, known as infodemics, which increased anxiety and made it difficult for individuals to make informed health decisions (Rathore & Farooq, 2020).

In addition, cultural differences in eating habits and medication preferences affected the health of those who had to be isolated and hospitalized. For example, some migrants preferred traditional medicines from their home countries, which they perceived as more effective than Japanese alternatives. The pandemic also highlighted issues of cultural appropriateness of healthcare services, such as dietary restrictions and the effectiveness of medications. Complaints were noted about the inadequacy of Japanese medicines, especially post-vaccination analgesics. Some residents, such as those in Nepal, preferred medicines from their own country, which they believed were more effective and were therefore imported privately. This phenomenon, deeply rooted in cultural familiarity and trust, suggests the need for more culturally sensitive medical practices. The information overload caused by the pandemic propagated through news, social media, and online sources, confused many people, and contributed to stress and anxiety. The rapid spread of misinformation and conspiracy theories (Rathore & Farooq, 2020) complicated the public's ability to trust health information and make informed decisions about vaccination and safety measures. In addition, the rise of telemedicine became a vital communication channel, especially for non-native speakers, facilitating access to health care and reducing the risk of infection. Telemedicine services for globally scattered Nepalese communities demonstrated how global homeland networks can support community health needs internationally.

Health centers played an important role in crisis management by conducting PCR testing, tracking contacts, and covering treatment costs. Japan's national health insurance system and other health services provided a positive incentive to visit clinics. On the other hand, challenges such as hospital opening times and the availability of medical interpreters remained, affecting the accessibility and quality of medical care received by foreign residents. These experiences underscore the need for a more comprehensive and adaptive Japanese healthcare system that addresses the linguistic and cultural barriers faced by foreign residents and utilizes modern technologies such as telemedicine to ensure equitable access to healthcare services. Healthcare policies and practices must reflect the diversity of the populations they serve to foster a healthier, more inclusive society.

Since the public health crisis of COVID-19 highlighted the critical challenges faced by migrants and the importance of ensuring timely access to health care for multilingual and multicultural communities and promoting a concerted global response, here we focus on the Nepalese migrants. The response of Nepalese migrants to COVID-19 in Japan is presented here as a case study. As of December 2023, Japan's resident foreign population is approximately 3,410,992, with the largest groups being Chinese, Vietnamese, Korean, Filipinos, Brazilians, and Nepalese (Immigration Services Agency of Japan, 2023). In response to the pandemic, the Ministry of Health, Labor and Welfare of Japan (MHLW) introduced a free 24-hour multilingual interpretation service, but as of October 2021, some languages remain unsupported. Although this service was essential to promoting better medical communication, barriers remain. Without adequate information and care, the migrants were increasingly vulnerable. There were very few Nepalese health workers in Japan, which further compounded the challenges faced by Nepalese migrants in accessing healthcare services and information. Recognizing this gap, a Nepalese nurse (the chapter author) took the initiative to spread awareness by creating informative videos about COVID-19 and sharing them on social networking sites (SNSs) in the local language.

Communication via Social Media Platforms Social networking sites (SNSs) such as TikTok, Facebook, and Instagram became crucial channels for communication. Numerous questions were asked, and there was a flood of messages seeking reliable information about COVID-19.

Creation of Informative TikTok Videos Frequently Asked Questions (FAQs) about COVID-19 were addressed through short, informative videos on TikTok. This platform was chosen for its wide reach and ease of sharing content.

Dissemination of Information Vital information about COVID-19, its symptoms, safety measures, data on recovery rates, the Japanese health care system, availability of healthcare services, vaccination information (different types of vaccines, eligibility criteria, and addressing rumors), mental health counseling, and home care management strategies was spread using SNS. The videos aimed to ensure accurate and up-to-date information to reach a broad audience within the Nepalese migrant community.

The response to these videos was overwhelming, with a significant increase in the number of followers, comments, and many migrants reaching out with calls, messages, and queries on social media platforms like Instagram and messengers. Recognizing the need for further support, the author collaborated with Japanese nurses to create additional videos on topics such as communicating in easy Japanese language, taking care of one's health at home, and identifying situations that require hospital visits. All the information was conveyed in the Nepalese language to ensure effective communication and understanding. The comments and feedback received from the viewers were overwhelmingly positive, with many expressing gratitude for the valuable information provided in their native language. This initiative not only helped bridge the information gap but also fostered a sense of community and support among the Nepalese migrants during a challenging time (Paudel & Kanbara, 2023).

This initiative during the COVID-19 pandemic can be regarded as a transformative nursing approach to addressing the challenges faced by the Nepalese migrant community in Japan, which not only bridged the information gap but also fostered a sense of community and support among the Nepalese migrants during a challenging time. The approach can be analyzed through the lens of three key aspects: data making, design thinking, and practical implementation (Fig. 4.2).

Data Making The overwhelming response from migrants, including the influx of calls, messages, and queries, highlighted the significant information gap and the need for tailored solutions. The nursing initiative inadvertently led to the collection of valuable data, which provided insights into the specific challenges and informa-

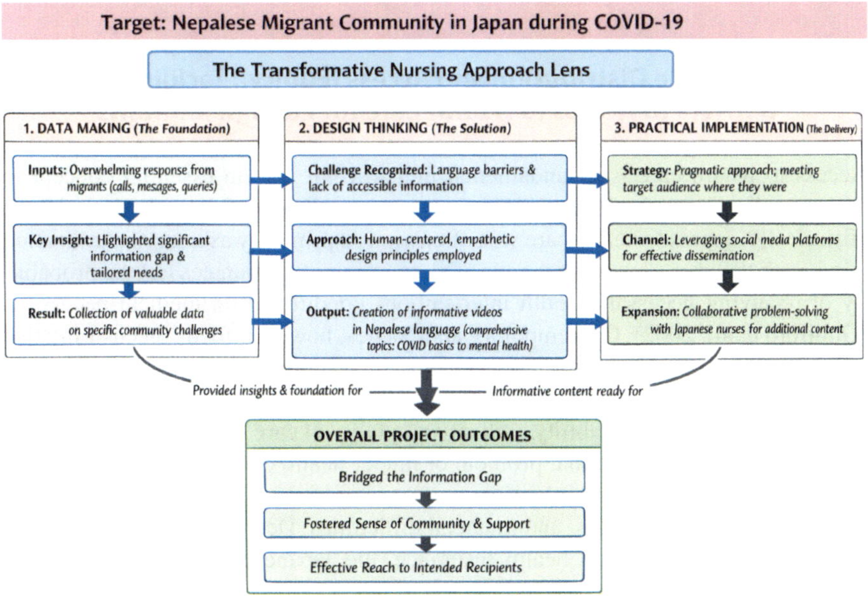

Fig. 4.2 A transformative nursing approach through three lenses

tion needs of the Nepalese migrant community. This data served as a foundation for developing targeted and effective solutions.

Design Thinking The nursing decision to create informative videos in the Nepalese language demonstrated a human-centered design approach. By recognizing the language barrier and the lack of accessible information, the nurse employed design thinking principles to develop a solution that addressed the unique needs of the target audience. The videos covered a comprehensive range of topics, from COVID-19 basics to mental health support, exhibiting a thoughtful and empathetic design process.

Practical Implementation The decision to leverage social media platforms as a means of disseminating the informative videos was a pragmatic and effective approach. By meeting the target audience where they were already present and engaged, the author ensured that the information reached the intended recipients effectively. Furthermore, the collaboration with Japanese nurses to create additional content demonstrated a collaborative approach to problem-solving and a commitment to providing comprehensive support.

4.5 Discussion Based on the Case Studies

Based on the above case studies, we will discuss the necessary initiatives for foreigners in the future based on the principles of PHC.

4.5.1 Equitable Distribution and Access (Equity): Tackling Barriers to Access to Health Care for Foreign Migrants

Access to health care is a fundamental human right and an essential concept in health policy and health services research (OHCHR, 2008; WHO, 2017). Historically, access to health care was often viewed primarily as a service utilization issue, with theories such as Shengelia et al. focusing on guarantees as "the probability of receiving necessary health interventions conditional on medical necessity" (Gulliford et al., 2002). Contemporary approaches, however, focus on ensuring that individuals have access to appropriate health care resources to maintain and improve their health. This includes considering availability, affordability, appropriateness, geographic access, acceptability, utilization, quality of care, and consumer satisfaction as interrelated factors that promote or hinder health care access. In Japan, foreign migrants face significant barriers to accessing health care, including language barriers, cultural differences, and financial difficulties. Despite the high standard of medical care and universal health insurance, the Japanese health care system is often inaccessible to those who do not speak Japanese or are unfamiliar with local medical practices. Language barriers are especially severe, hindering effective communication regarding medical procedures and symptoms. Not only does this hinder accurate diagnosis and treatment, but it also affects their ability to successfully navigate the healthcare system, such as making appointments and understanding referrals.

The cultural nuances of the Japanese healthcare system, often accompanied by indirect communication styles and conservative discussions of medical prognosis, are incredibly challenging for foreigners accustomed to more straightforward communication. Such cultural gaps can lead to misunderstandings, dissatisfaction with the care received, non-adherence to medical advice, and worse health outcomes.

Furthermore, many foreign migrants come from countries where healthcare systems are less robust and systematic than in Japan. They may be overwhelmed by the complexity and sophistication of Japanese medical facilities, especially when they require specific medical specialties or advanced treatments. In addition, access to such specialized medical care is expensive and rare. Furthermore, many cultures rely on home remedies or wait for symptoms rather than seek medical advice. The lack of access to appropriate medical care abroad compounds this trend. Japanese healthcare providers are encouraged to further enhance their cultural competence in order to effectively respond to the needs of an increasingly diverse population. This includes language support through interpreters and multilingual resources and a deeper understanding of the diverse medical beliefs and practices of different cultures. Institutional changes are also needed to ensure that migrants have better access to medical care, including more comprehensive health care policies, improved patient education, and community support programs that address the foreign population's practical and cultural needs. Thus, addressing inequities in access to health care for foreign migrants in Japan is critical not only for the well-being of this vulnerable population but also for the integrity and effectiveness of the health care system. Increasing equity in access to health care requires a better understanding of the diverse needs of all populations and the coordination of services to meet these needs effectively and respectfully.

4.5.2 Strengthening Citizen Participation: Involvement of Foreign Residents in Community Activity Planning

Encouraging the participation of foreign residents in community activities is a necessary step toward a more comprehensive and effective public health strategy that goes beyond simply strengthening Japan's healthcare system. As Japan becomes more culturally diverse, including foreign immigrants in community planning activities is critical to developing a truly comprehensive public health framework. Ensuring that foreign residents are recipients of health care services and participants is essential for a democratic society to function effectively and promote an inclusive living environment. While this integration can enrich the experiences of foreign migrants, strengthen Japan's overall social fabric, and better respond to the country's evolving demographics, improved language services and cultural competence of health care providers are needed to facilitate this participation. Cultural background significantly influences health beliefs and practices, affecting health-seeking behaviors and perceptions of health care. Training health care providers in cultural competence is essential to reduce misconceptions and provide targeted assistance to people of diverse backgrounds. This includes involving foreign residents in assessments, program planning, and policymaking processes. Viewing established communities not merely as target groups but as platforms for voicing concerns and contributing insights can address specific health issues and foster a sense of local belonging among foreign migrants. These improvements are necessary for foreign residents to seek appropriate treatment or access health services, leading to misdiagnosis and inappropriate treatment, compromising patient safety and quality of care.

Organizational barriers often inhibit foreign migrants from participating, but their involvement in local policymaking ensures that their needs and perspectives are considered and addressed. For example, regular promotion of multicultural community development can lead to mutual assistance during a disaster. By providing appropriate information to foreign residents, they can take the same self-help and mutual-help actions as Japanese residents in emergencies. It is also essential to raise awareness of disaster prevention and provide opportunities to learn about it regularly. Even healthy people may face unforeseen difficulties during emergencies, and awareness of vulnerable populations can lead to proactive safety measures. During the public health crisis of COVID-19, collaboration among international students across various disciplines highlighted a coordinated approach to addressing the health and legal challenges migrants face. Unlike natural disasters, the global nature of the pandemic allowed anyone to access health services and consult with health care providers at any time and from any place through online platforms, reducing potential health disparities. Mutual aid is crucial in minimizing the impact of disasters. Mutual aid can be strengthened by expanding the role of foreign personnel, including nurses and doctors. These personnel can serve as essential volunteers and influencers and have the potential to effectively disseminate necessary information across different age groups and cultural backgrounds.

4.5.3 Multisectoral Collaboration: Integrating Public Services for Foreign Migrants

Effective integration and support of foreign residents in Japan requires a cohesive and comprehensive approach that transcends traditional sectoral boundaries. Multisectoral cooperation, including health care, education, communications, and local government, is essential to comprehensively address foreign residents' complex and intertwined needs. This collaboration is essential to improve medical care and disaster preparedness and adequately address all aspects of migrants' lives, including legal assistance, employment, and social integration.

Foreign migrants often face challenges beyond health care, such as legal problems, employment barriers, and social integration difficulties. Each of these factors significantly impacts their overall well-being and ability to thrive in their new environment. For example, unfamiliarity with the legal system can lead to exploitation and inadequate protection in the workplace. At the same time, difficulties with social integration can exacerbate feelings of isolation and stress, which can further affect mental health, especially during disasters. A strategic administrative framework is needed to integrate services between different sectors. There is a need to establish a formal organization that brings together representatives from health, education, employment, housing, and social services. This body will develop policies and programs that comprehensively address the needs of migrants and ensure the coordination of existing policies to effectively support foreign residents. For example, after the Great Hanshin-Awaji Earthquake, Kobe City started to create soil to accept internationalization, made many efforts in disaster prevention, and established the Medical Industry City and the Health Creation City. The "Regional Collaboration Bureau," newly established through organizational reform, conducted detailed hearings and surveys in the community. Through the hearings and surveys, many issues were brought to light. By sharing regional issues and future visions with various residents, including citizens, neighborhood associations, NPOs, and businesses, the bureau promotes community development by taking advantage of their expertise and sharing roles and responsibilities (Kobe Biomedical Innovation Cluster, 2022).

Setting up a familiar consultation service for daily life, such as health and legal services, is also necessary. The activities of the "Town Health Room," a volunteer group of the Nursing Association that began after the Great Hanshin-Awaji Earthquake, and consultations with NPOs have revealed that foreign residents face language barriers, cultural differences, and a lack of information on medical and welfare services. As a result, they may be unable to pay medical bills or experience increased stress at work and in their daily lives. As observed during the COVID-19 pandemic and in other situations, migrants' access to medical care is often compromised by language barriers, financial difficulties, and lack of multilingual translation services at health centers. In addition, migrants are often accused and stigmatized for spreading disease; effective collaboration and advocacy with NGOs and support groups, fundraising, cultural competency education for health care providers, and building trust and familiarity are essential facilitators for improving access to health and social services for foreign migrants (Edward & Hines-Martin, 2014). Thus, by integrating services across health, education, employment, and social sectors, Japan can not only improve health outcomes for migrants but also promote integration within public policy and enrich the broader community. Such a holistic approach is a critical issue not only for foreign migrants but also for the inclusiveness of social and economic health in the country as a whole.

4.5.4 Appropriate Technology: Improving Accessibility for Foreign Migrants Through Digital Solutions

Digital solutions have emerged as powerful tools to enhance healthcare accessibility for foreign migrants, particularly those facing language barriers or unfamiliarity with local healthcare systems. Telemedicine services offering consultations in multiple languages can enable timely medical advice and treatment without the need for in-person visits, thereby reducing barriers to care. Such services are especially beneficial for individuals who might otherwise delay seeking help due to communication challenges or logistical difficulties. Alongside telemedicine, investments in health data analytics can yield significant benefits. By leveraging technology to collect and analyze health-related data, foreign residents can gain insights into their specific health trends and needs. Moreover, big data analytics can monitor broader health impacts of environmental changes and disasters, facilitating targeted public health responses and optimized resource allocation. This data-driven approach not only improves individual care but also strengthens systemic resilience.

However, the implementation of these technological solutions must be thoughtfully executed to ensure inclusivity. It is crucial that digital health platforms are well-designed and accessible to all segments of the foreign population, including those with varying levels of technological literacy or access. Failing to address the digital divide risks exacerbating existing inequalities rather than mitigating them. Several challenges accompany the integration of technology in health care, including privacy concerns, the aforementioned digital divide, and the costs associated with developing and maintaining high-quality digital health services. To overcome these hurdles, robust privacy protections must be established to safeguard sensitive health information. Efforts to increase digital literacy among foreign residents are also essential, as are sustainable financing models to support ongoing technological innovation and maintenance.

4.5.5 Building Knowledge and Capacity: Strengthening Training Programs for Diversity and Inclusive Health and Disaster Management

The imperative for robust training programs addressing the health needs of vulnerable populations, such as foreign residents in Japan, has become increasingly apparent. These initiatives must transcend mere medical knowledge, encompassing culturally appropriate care and services tailored to diverse populations, with considerations for age, gender, literacy levels, and myriad other factors that influence health outcomes and service utilization. In an era of heightened globalization and migration, healthcare providers increasingly encounter patients from diverse cultural and ethnic backgrounds, each bringing unique perspectives on health, illness, and treatment. Migrants often exhibit varied cultural reactions to Western medicine, which can profoundly impact their healthcare utilization patterns. A frequently cited socio-cultural and economic barrier is the disparity stemming from differences in healthcare systems between their countries of origin and their new home. The COVID-19 pandemic starkly illuminated how these cultural barriers can exacerbate stress among migrants, sometimes manifesting as hesitancy toward preventive measures like vaccination.

Furthermore, health outcomes are influenced by factors such as length of stay and reason for entry, underscoring the need for nuanced, context-specific approaches.

Traditional information dissemination methods—word of mouth, email, or paper-based materials—have shown limitations in reaching foreign residents effectively. Paper-based information, in particular, suffers from inflexibility in updates and distribution scope. This highlights the necessity of devising strategies to make people aware of and overcome invisible barriers to information access, especially in areas with significant foreign resident populations. Collaboration with workplaces and educational institutions that have large numbers of foreign residents may prove instrumental in communicating critical health and safety information. The legal framework regulating access to resources such as health insurance and medical care also plays a pivotal role in health outcomes. For instance, in communities with substantial first-generation refugee populations, like the Indochinese community in Japan, many have adapted to local norms, including language proficiency, which aids in daily interactions and service access. However, even long-term, Japanese-speaking residents may face inadequate access to medical services due to institutional barriers and a lack of culturally appropriate healthcare provision.

Given these complexities, training programs must be comprehensive, addressing not only medical knowledge but also cultural competence, legal rights awareness, and communication skills. These programs should be dynamic, incorporating feedback from both healthcare providers and foreign residents to ensure relevance and responsiveness to changing needs and emerging health issues in migrant populations. Training methodologies should be diverse, including case studies, role-playing exercises, and partnerships with migrant communities to guarantee effectiveness and pertinence. The establishment of such robust training programs is critical for building the capacity of healthcare providers to meet the needs of diverse populations competently and sensitively. These efforts should aim to improve medical outcomes for foreign residents, enhance the professional development of healthcare providers, and foster a more empathetic, informed, and responsive healthcare environment in Japan. The benefits of this approach extend beyond the medical field, contributing to the broader integration and social inclusion of migrants into Japanese society.

4.5.6 Securing Resources for Integrated Health and Social Programs

The social determinants of health—encompassing the conditions in which people are born, grow, live, work, and age—are profoundly shaped by the distribution of money, power, and resources. Addressing these determinants necessitates a collaborative, cross-sectoral approach. Integrated financing, which coordinates investments across multiple sectors, has emerged as a powerful strategy to improve population health and promote health equity. This approach is particularly potent in tackling complex health problems rooted in multifaceted social and environmental factors. Economic barriers frequently impede access to health services, with high costs serving as a significant risk factor for adverse health outcomes. For migrants in Japan, especially those supporting family members abroad, economic constraints can severely hamper access to health care, often delaying necessary treatment due to the prohibitive cost of medical services. Despite Japan's universal health insurance system, which ostensibly reduces healthcare costs, surveys have revealed that a lack of awareness about health insurance coverage remains a substantial barrier. Alarmingly, more than half of respondents report not visiting hospitals, perceiving medical care as expensive and only available when symptoms are apparent, often unaware of the benefits to which they are entitled. Another economic hurdle is the lack of price transparency, which discourages individuals from seeking medical care due to the specter of unexpected expenses. This issue was prominently noted in one study, where uncertainty about healthcare costs led many to forego needed medical services. During the COVID-19 crisis, the need for frequent examinations posed a financial challenge not only for migrants but also for the government, reflecting the broader economic ramifications of health emergencies.

In light of these challenges, it is imperative to empower communities to allocate funds according to local health and social needs and to increase the effectiveness and transparency of resource use. Such measures would foster community participation in budgetary decisions and enhance the credibility and accountability of health activities. A comprehensive strategy that understands the context of Primary Health Care (PHC), including the needs of foreign migrants, is essential for integrating health with other vital sectors to address the wide range of social determinants affecting health. The reorganization of financial support mechanisms should aim to improve the accessibility and quality of healthcare for all residents, with a particular focus on foreign residents. This involves ensuring that the healthcare system is inclusive, equitable, and adaptable to the increasingly diverse needs of the population. To alleviate economic barriers, expanding eligibility for national health insurance coverage and providing accessible, multilingual information on health insurance utilization are critical steps toward a comprehensive healthcare system. These measures, coupled with efforts to increase price transparency and community involvement in resource allocation, can significantly reduce disparities in healthcare access and outcomes.

4.6 Conclusion and Future Directions

Japan is experiencing a significant influx of foreign residents, a trend that brings to the fore pressing concerns about their health and safety, particularly in the face of potential major disasters that could have devastating consequences. As a host to a substantial number of foreign nationals, Japan must anticipate and address escalating apprehensions regarding the well-being of new immigrants, especially during crises or disasters. The presence of foreign nurses and doctors in Japan represents a vital volunteer resource capable of saving lives—both native and non-native—underscoring the importance of inclusive disaster preparedness and response strategies. The media emerges as an influential stakeholder in disaster risk reduction, bearing the responsibility of effectively disseminating reliable and essential information. In this age of infodemic, the challenge lies in ensuring that critical information reaches diverse age groups and cultural backgrounds, necessitating culturally sensitive communication strategies. Concurrently, the optimization of global telemedicine services dedicated to addressing health issues specific to one's home country presents a promising avenue. Such services could be particularly beneficial for those facing language barriers when visiting healthcare facilities and could prove invaluable during crises. Referral healthcare facilities leveraging telemedicine can enhance patient safety and quality of care, bridging gaps in accessibility. A critical issue is the lack of awareness among migrants about Japan's universal healthcare system, contributing to their higher morbidity rates compared to nationals. For universal healthcare to fulfill its mandate, no one must be left behind. This calls for innovative approaches, such as making documentation and information on health insurance mandatory at the time of visa issuance, akin to requirements for visas, travel insurance, and vaccine passports. The bureaucratic hurdles often encountered during crises, causing delays in service delivery, can be mitigated through alternative and flexible policies.

Furthermore, strengthening mutual aid within communities during peacetime can illuminate the reasons, barriers, and facilitators preventing priority populations from accessing or benefiting from services. True disaster reduction transcends the mere provision of supplies and temporary assistance; it is achieved when people collaborate and learn to enrich their lives and ensure their safety independently. This process fosters understanding between residents and foreigners of each other's thoughts, values, and customs—a critical step toward creating a more secure community.

Japan's Ministry of Internal Affairs and Communications (MIC) has emphasized the importance of multicultural conviviality, where people of different nationalities and ethnicities coexist as equal members of the local community while acknowledging cultural differences. Local governments, confronted with tangible issues such as education and medical care for foreign residents, have often pioneered efforts toward multicultural conviviality ahead of national initiatives, embodying this philosophy in practice.

Leveraging daily touchpoints such as schools, train stations, and other frequented locales as information hubs is considered a strategic shortcut from community-level information exchange to region-wide dissemination. This approach recognizes the power of integrating critical information into the fabric of daily life. Based on these insights, it is imperative to enhance disaster prevention education and refine information provision methods in Japan. Promoting efforts that enable foreigners to live safely and comfortably in Japan is not just a matter of crisis management but a fundamental aspect of building an inclusive, resilient society. The path forward demands a multifaceted approach: harnessing technology to bridge communication gaps, embedding health and safety awareness into the immigration process, fostering community-led support systems, and cultivating a culture of mutual understanding and respect. By prioritizing these elements, Japan can work toward a future where every resident, regardless of origin, feels secure, valued, and prepared in the face of adversity. This vision of inclusive disaster preparedness and healthcare accessibility is not only a moral imperative but also a strategic necessity in our increasingly interconnected world.

Study Guide Questions

These questions are designed to help readers—whether you are a practicing Advanced Practice Nurse (APN) at Level III, aspiring to this role, or supporting competency development in disaster nursing—apply concepts from this chapter to real-world practice. Each question aligns with specific ICN Disaster Nursing Core Competency domains and emphasizes transcultural nursing, Primary Health Care principles, and Open Governance in multicultural disaster contexts.

Questions

1. *Domain 1 (Preparation and Planning) and Domain 8 (Law and Ethics)*:
   Drawing from this chapter's discussion of Open Governance and the four-domain framework of healthcare access barriers (Table 4.1), design a comprehensive disaster preparedness plan for your community that addresses the needs of foreign residents. How would you integrate the concepts of cultural competence, cultural humility, and transcultural nursing into this plan? Consider legal frameworks, ethical principles of equity, and the PHC pillars discussed in this chapter (equity, civic participation, multisectoral collaboration, and appropriate technology).
2. *Domain 2 (Communication) and Domain 4 (Safety and Security)*:
   This chapter describes the Nepalese nurse's experience creating COVID-19 information resources in 11 languages and managing an overwhelming community response. Evaluate multilingual communication systems in your organization or community using the Healthcare Access Barriers Framework presented in this chapter. What specific improvements would you propose in each of the four domains (availability and accommodation, affordability, adequacy, and acceptability)? How would you balance technological solutions with human-centered approaches?
3. *Domain 5 (Assessment) and Domain 6 (Intervention)*:
   Reflecting on the case studies presented (Nepalese nurse case study, experiences during the Great East Japan Earthquake, and COVID-19 responses), develop a culturally sensitive assessment protocol for foreign residents in disaster contexts. How would you operationalize Leininger's Culture Care Theory (culture care preservation, accommodation, and repatterning) in your assessment and intervention strategies? What specific cultural adaptations would be necessary in your local context?
4. *Domain 3 (Incident Management) and Domain 7 (Recovery)*:
   This chapter discusses the transformation of PHC required by future society and emphasizes mutual aid over one-directional support. Design a post-disaster recovery plan that operationalizes the six PHC principles discussed (equitable distribution and access, civic participation, multisectoral collaboration, appropriate technology, knowledge and capacity building, and human resources for

health). How would you ensure that foreign residents transition from being "supported" to being active partners in community recovery?

5. *Professional Leadership and Cross-Cultural Competency Development*:
   Consider this chapter's discussion of transcultural nursing as an operational bridge between PHC and disaster response. How would you develop and evaluate a training program that moves nurses through the three phases of gender awareness transformation (gender blind → gender aware → gender transformative) while integrating cultural competence and cultural humility? What pedagogical methods would be most effective for developing these competencies in Level I and II nurses?
6. *Systems Thinking and Policy Integration*:
   This chapter positions multicultural community care as a practical test of Open Governance. Analyze how the concepts of "Jimoto" (home community) and "Sosei" (creation/revitalization) can be integrated into disaster risk reduction policy in your jurisdiction. What systemic barriers exist to implementing truly participatory, multicultural disaster preparedness? How would you advocate for policy changes that promote health equity for foreign residents?

Acknowledgments The authors thank Seiko Iimura (research assistant, Kobe City College of Nursing) for her editorial support and literature coordination. Generative AI tools were used to assist with drafting and language refinement; all content was critically reviewed and approved by the authors. The authors are grateful to the multicultural communities in Kochi Prefecture whose lived experiences of navigating health and social services informed the perspectives in this chapter.

Author Contributions Conceptualization: Sushila Paudel, Sakiko Kanbara. Writing—original draft: Sushila Paudel; editorial coordination by Sakiko Kanbara. Writing—review and editing: Sakiko Kanbara; editorial and linguistic assistance provided by a research assistant (Seiko Iimura). Literature search and reference management: Research assistant (Seiko Iimura). AI-assisted drafting: Generative AI tools were used to support initial structuring and language refinement under the supervision of the authors.

Definitions

Migrant/foreign resident: A person living in the host country with a foreign nationality under a range of residence statuses (e.g., worker, student, family). In this chapter, we use "foreign resident" in line with Immigration Services Agency (ISA) foreign resident statistics.

Access to health care: A multi-dimensional concept that goes beyond "service use," including availability, affordability, acceptability, and quality from the user perspective (Gulliford et al., 2002).

Health equity (and inequity): Equity refers to fair opportunities to attain the highest possible level of health; inequities are systematic, avoidable differences in health outcomes and in the conditions that shape them (Marmot, 2007).

Transcultural nursing/culturally congruent care: A nursing approach that aims to provide care that fits patients' cultural values, beliefs, and lifeways in ways that are meaningful and beneficial (Leininger, 2002).

Primary Health Care (PHC) and mutual aid: PHC is a people-centered approach to health that emphasizes equity, community participation, multisectoral action, and appropriate technology; mutual aid highlights residents' capacity to act together rather than being treated only as recipients of support (WHO, 2017).

Disaster risk reduction (DRR): A systematic approach to reducing disaster risks by preventing new risks, reducing existing risks, and strengthening preparedness, including the strengthening of disaster risk governance (UNDRR, 2015).

References

Bahar, A., Koçak, H. S., Samancıoğlu Bağlama, S., & Çuhadar, D. (2020). Can psychological resilience protect the mental health of healthcare professionals during the COVID-19 pandemic period? *Dubai Medical Journal, 3*(4), 133–139.

Barış, E., Silverman, R., Wang, H., & Zhao, F. (2022). *Walking the talk: Reimagining primary health care after COVID-19*. World Bank Publications.

Blomberg, B., Mohn, K. G. I., Brokstad, K. A., Zhou, F., Linchausen, D. W., Hansen, B. A., et al. (2021). Long COVID in a prospective cohort of home-isolated patients. *Nature Medicine, 27*(9), 1607–1613.

Council of Local Authorities for International Relations (CLAIR). (2024). *Multiculturalism promotion*. https://www.clair.or.jp/e/multiculture/tagengo/preparing-for-a-natural-disaster.html

Edward, J., & Hines-Martin, V. (2014). Exploring the providers perspective of health and social service availability for immigrants and refugees in a southern urban community. *Journal of Immigrant and Minority Health, 17*(4), 1185–1191.

Germain, S., & Yong, A. (2020). COVID-19 highlighting inequalities in access to healthcare in England: A case study of ethnic minority and migrant women. *Feminist Legal Studies, 28*(3), 301–310.

Guadagno, L. (2020). *Migrants and the COVID-19 pandemic: An initial analysis*. https://publications.iom.int/system/files/pdf/mrs-60.pdf

Gulliford, M., Figueroa-Munoz, J., Morgan, M., Hughes, D., Gibson, B., Beech, R., & Hudson, M. (2002). What does 'access to health care' mean? *Journal of Health Services Research & Policy, 7*(3), 186–188.

Immigration Service Agency. (2025). *Number of foreign residents in Japan*. https://www.moj.go.jp/isa/content/001447921.pdf. Accessed 30 Apr 2025.

Immigration Services Agency of Japan. (2023). *Foreign resident statistics*. https://www.moj.go.jp/isa/content/001447921.pdf.

Immigration Services Agency of Japan. (2025). *Foreign resident statistics*. https://www.moj.go.jp/isa/content/001434755.pdf. Accessed 30 Apr 2025.

International Council of Nurses. (2021). *The ICN code of ethics for nurses*. https://www.icn.ch/sites/default/files/2023-06/ICN_Code-of-Ethics_EN_Web.pdf

IOM. (2011). *Handbook for migrants vulnerable to violence, exploitation, and abuse on protection and assistance*. Retrieved from website: https://publications.iom.int/system/files/pdf/avm_handbook.pdf

Kobe Biomedical Innovation Cluster. (2022). https://www.fbri-kobe.org/kbic/english/movies/download/kbic_attract_eng2022.pdf. Accessed 30 Apr 2025.

Koh, D. (2020). Migrant workers and COVID-19. *Occupational and Environmental Medicine, 77*(9), 634–636. https://doi.org/10.1136/oemed-2020-106626. Accessed 30 Apr 2025.

Lebano, A., Hamed, S., Bradby, H., Gil-Salmerón, A., Durá-Ferrandis, E., Garcés-Ferrer, J., & Linos, A. (2020). Migrants' and refugees' health status and healthcare in Europe: A scoping literature review. *BMC Public Health, 20*(1). https://doi.org/10.1186/s12889-020-08749-8. Accessed 30 Apr 2025.

Leininger, M. (2002). Culture care theory: A major contribution to advance transcultural nursing knowledge and practices. *Journal of Transcultural Nursing, 13*(3), 189–192.

Marmot, M. (2007). Achieving health equity: From root causes to fair outcomes. *The Lancet, 370*(9593), 1153–1163.

Ochi, S., Murray, V., & Hodgson, S. (2013). The great East Japan earthquake disaster: A compilation of published literature on health needs and relief activities, March 2011–September 2012. *PLoS Currents*. Vol.5, 1–37, https://doi.org/10.1371/currents.dis.771beae7d8f41c31cd91e765678c005d

OECD. (2021). *Realising the potential of primary health care. OECD health policy studies*. OECD Publishing. https://doi.org/10.1787/a92adee4-en

OHCHR. (2008). *Principles and guidelines migrants in vulnerable situations, supported by practical guidance, on the human rights protection of migrants in vulnerable situations*. Retrieved from website: https://www.ohchr.org/Documents/Issues/Migration/PrinciplesAndGuidelines.pdf. Accessed 30 Apr 2025.

Paudel, S., & Kanbara, S. (2023). Enhancing healthcare access during disasters and emergencies: Recommendations from Nepali migrants in Japan. *Dialogues Health, 6*(2), 100136. https://doi.org/10.1016/j.dialog.2023.100136. PMID: 38515473; PMCID: PMC10953979.

Rathore, F. A., & Farooq, F. (2020). Information overload and infodemic in the COVID-19 pandemic. *The Journal of the Pakistan Medical Association, 70*(5), S162–S165.

Science Council of Japan. (2013). *Proposals from the academic community.—Now, let us take strong steps toward recovery—*. https://www.scj.go.jp/ja/info/kohyo/pdf/kohyo-22-t-shien1.pdf. Accessed 30 Apr 2025.

Shah, M. F., & Murao, O. (2013). Foreigners' evacuation behavior in the Great East Japan earthquake: A case of Iwaki City in Fukushima Prefecture. *Journal of Disaster Research, 8*(sp), 802–813. https://doi.org/10.20965/jdr.2013.p0802. Accessed 30 Apr 2025.

UNDRR. (2015). *What is Sendai Framework?* https://www.undrr.org/implementing-sendai-framework/what-sendai-framework

WHO. (2017). *Human rights and health*. Retrieved June 29, 2021, from Who.int. https://www.who.int/news-room/fact-sheets/detail/human-rights-and-health. Accessed 30 Apr 2025.

5 Empowering Rural Health Systems: Integrative Digital Strategies for Enhanced Community Well-Being

Yuri Machida, Megumi Fujii, and Sakiko Kanbara

5.1 Introduction

The World Health Organization's (WHO) Global Strategy for People-Centred Integrated Health Services 2016–2026 advocates health services that put the preferences and needs of individuals, families, and communities at the center (WHO, 2015). Promoting Digital Integration at the Local Level To successfully digitize community health services, it is crucial to implement information technology (IT) solutions that meet the community's specific needs. This includes developing and implementing digital tools tailored to enhance health service delivery and community participation.

Japan is facing rapid and profound demographic changes, more severe than in many other countries, characterized by population decline and aging. In response, under its Fifth Science and Technology Basic Plan, the Japanese government has set forth the "Society 5.0" vision (Cabinet Office, 2021). This vision aims to foster a resilient and sustainable society amidst myriad threats and uncertainties, ensuring every citizen's security and diverse well-being. The COVID-19 pandemic has highlighted these flaws and spurred the adoption and advancement of 5G, IoT, and AI technologies. One of its most ubiquitous connected tools, the smartphone, has revolutionized access to vast information and knowledge worldwide. Over the past two decades, smartphone penetration has skyrocketed in mainstream consumer markets worldwide. These devices have become extremely important in our daily lives,

Y. Machida
Peace Winds Japan, Kochi, Japan

F. Fujii
Faculty of Nursing, Japanese Red Cross Toyota College of Nursing, Toyota, Japan

M. Kanbara (✉)
Faculty of Nursing, Kobe City College of Nursing, Kobe, Japan
e-mail: s-kanbara@kobe-ccn.ac.jp

S. Kanbara (ed.), *Transformative Community Health Nursing*,
https://doi.org/10.1007/978-3-032-24405-5_5

impacting areas ranging from business to education. Expanding the hardware and software markets associated with smartphones is a significant economic driver. At the individual level, smartphones have been shown to reduce stress in hectic work environments and serve as a source of healthcare through various applications.

With this progress, challenges remain in laying a solid foundation for current initiatives to be developed as sustainable policies. According to a METI study, for digital health solutions to be effective and sustainable, they must address a wide range of community needs. Ongoing policy evaluation and adaptation are necessary to respond to changing community needs. Such a dynamic approach will ensure that health services remain relevant and effective in addressing personal-community-specific health challenges (METI, 2020). Digitalization of community services and capacity building in the community are essential to sustain digital initiatives. This requires educating residents on digital competencies and establishing a framework for cooperation between local and external human resources based on trust and mutual understanding. The participation of various stakeholders is essential and is vital to align community goals with the capabilities of digital health solution providers to ensure the continued delivery of needed services. This includes integrating these solutions into the broader community health infrastructure and adapting to changing local conditions. Partnership building among municipalities, healthcare providers, technology experts, and community organizations to eliminate health inequities is also necessary to develop health services. These collaborations should focus on building integrated, people-centered health systems that reflect the principles of equity, human rights, and gender equality advocated in the WHO's Global Strategy. Emphasize open governance so that all community members, especially the vulnerable and elderly, can participate in decision-making. Integrating smartphones and extensive digital infrastructure into daily life can bridge these gaps and provide new avenues for enhancing the well-being of all citizens, especially the elderly.

There, we aim to provide a concise and clear introduction to the topics covered in the book, setting the stage for a more in-depth look at the impact of smartphone adoption among the elderly in Japan and its broader implications for health care and social inclusion. By adopting these recommendations, similar communities can build strong, equitable, and innovative health systems that can respond to the rapid changes and challenges of the digital age, ultimately leading to improved health outcomes and quality of life for the community.

5.2 Impact of Smartphones on the Elderly

Smartphones' rapid development and proliferation have intensified a longstanding issue: the digital divide. The World Economic Forum, in its Global Risks Report 2021, highlights the barriers to digital inclusivity as one of the most significant risks, particularly as nations increasingly grapple with aging populations (The World Economic Forum, 2021). This digital divide, defined by Rowena Cullen in 2001, exists between those with ready access to information and communication technologies and the knowledge they offer and those without (Cullen, 2001). Initially, the digital divide was seen predominantly as a gap between developed and developing regions. However, as smartphones have become primary internet access tools, the divide between generations, especially between the elderly and younger populations, has become more pronounced.

This growth is mirrored in developed nations; in the United States, 42% of those over 65 owned smartphones in 2017, up from 18% in 2013 (Anderson & Perrin, 2017). In the UK, 67% of the elderly reported using a smartphone in 2022, a significant increase from 28% in 2015 (Laricchia, 2024). In China, the proportion of elderly internet users has been growing. In 2021, about 130 million older adults used smartphones to access the internet, representing more than 49% of the elderly population (CNNIC, 2021). Data from Japan clearly shows this gap: while over 90% of internet users aged 20–39 use their smartphones as their primary internet devices, less than 40% of those aged 70–80 do so (MIC, 2021). This disparity indicates a severe digital divide, which could lead to inequalities in access to critical information, such as real-time updates, during natural disasters—a common occurrence in Japan. Therefore, addressing smartphone penetration among the elderly is crucial to narrowing this digital divide.

5.2.1 Conceptual Pathway: Digital Divide, Health Inequity, and Disaster Risk Reduction (DRR)

To make the underlying logic explicit, Rad presents a simple causal pathway showing how the digital divide can translate into health inequity and, in disaster-prone contexts, elevated disaster risk (Rad, 2025). Building on Cullen's definition of the digital divide as unequal access to information and communication technologies (ICT) and the knowledge they provide (Cullen, 2001), and the World Economic Forum's framing of barriers to digital inclusivity as a major global risk in aging societies, the model links national-level age-stratified smartphone usage data to community-level health and DRR outcomes. This conceptual framework illustrates how digital exclusion functions as a social determinant of health, systematically disadvantaging older adults in rural communities and increasing their vulnerability during disasters. Understanding this causal pathway is essential for designing effective interventions that address not only the technological gap but also the underlying health inequities it perpetuates.

In later sections, the Hidaka Village initiative is presented as a practical approach to interrupt this pathway by strengthening capacity (digital literacy and social support), improving access (infrastructure and affordability), and institutionalizing people-centered governance and continuous evaluation.

Globally, efforts to bridge the digital divide for older adults are reshaping their quality of life and enhancing their welfare. Research has shown that internet use can significantly benefit the psychological health of older adults. For example, studies by Shaw L. H. and Gant L. M. have demonstrated that internet use can decrease social isolation and depression and enhance users' perceptions of social support and self-esteem (Shaw & Gant, 2002). These benefits are particularly poignant for the elderly, who may use technology to maintain connections, access entertainment, and manage health information more independently. However, the internet also presents challenges for the elderly, such as navigating user interfaces that are not elder-friendly or overcoming the fear of technology. These issues underscore the necessity for targeted training and support to help older adults become comfortable and proficient with digital technology. At this stage, the rise of smartphones is bringing new social challenges while also solving new ones, such as the shrinking PC market and the increase in smartphone addiction, negatively affecting the educational environment and health (Sarwar & Soomro, 2013). According to the Ministry of Internal Affairs and Communications' 2020 survey, smartphone ownership has increased to 86.8% of households and 69.3% of individuals. However, there is a significant disparity in ownership rates among the elderly, especially those in their 70s and 80s, compared to other age groups (MIC, 2021). Like many other aging societies, Japan is grappling with these issues, but the dual arrival of an aging and digital society presents both challenges and opportunities. Integrating the elderly into the digital world involves providing the necessary tools and technologies and ensuring they have the skills and support to use them effectively. This includes designing user-friendly interfaces, offering personalized training, and creating community programs encouraging digital participation. By addressing these areas, society can help bridge the digital divide and ensure that older adults are included in our rapidly evolving digital world.

5.3 Case Study 1: Hidaka Village

Effective integration of smartphones into the lives of elderly residents requires a nuanced understanding of their daily routines and social structures. Adoption is facilitated more smoothly by aligning smartphone functionalities with the villagers' lifestyles and interests. For instance, integrating health monitoring apps or easy communication tools like WhatsApp has shown potential. Encouraging smartphones within existing community groups and activities helps demonstrate their practical benefits in real-time, leading to more organic growth in acceptance and use.

One illustrative example of these efforts is found in Hidaka Village, Kochi Prefecture. Here, the local government has launched an ambitious initiative to digitize the entire village, promoting community-wide adoption of smartphones as a first step toward this futuristic vision. Overcoming the challenges associated with introducing smartphones to elderly populations in rural settings like Hidaka Village requires addressing tangible barriers, such as cost and usability, as well as intangible ones, like a perceived necessity. By tailoring approaches that consider the unique lifestyles and community dynamics of the elderly, Hidaka Village is making meaningful progress toward digital inclusivity (Hidaka Village, 2021).

Hidaka Village, nestled among mountains and rivers and approximately 40 min by car from central Kochi Prefecture, has experienced a significant demographic shift. Since reaching a peak population of 7926 in 1954, the village has steadily declined in residents, particularly among the younger, child-rearing demographic. As of April 2020, the village population was 4746, with 2066 residents aged 65 and over, marking an aging rate of 43.7% (Kochi Prefecture, 2021). The village has actively sought to counter these trends by welcoming immigrants from other prefectures, bolstering support for child-rearing, and promoting local industries. A notable historical challenge for Hidaka Village has been its vulnerability to floods, particularly severe events in 1975 and 1976. These events underscored the need for a robust communication infrastructure. In response, early initiatives included the installation of optical fiber cables throughout the village and dedicated communication equipment, establishing a resilient network foundation that would later support its digital transformation.

The digital divide between generations was evident in Hidaka Village. While younger generations grow up with technology, many elderly residents have spent most of their lives without digital devices. This generational gap influences how different age groups perceive and interact with technology.

Tailoring smartphone functionalities to fit the lifestyles and interests of the elderly was essential for effective health promotion and increased well-being within the community. Promoting the security and benefits of digital tools can help overcome the psychological barriers many older adults face regarding technology adoption. Smartphones could be a crucial link between the elderly and healthcare services, especially in areas with limited physical healthcare infrastructure. Apps that monitor health metrics and provide virtual consultations can improve access to care and health literacy among the elderly. Moreover, integrating smartphones into community activities could strengthen social connections and reduce feelings of isolation. Smartphones can help the elderly feel more included in society and increase their engagement with the community and family, leading to improved mental health and well-being.

Efforts to overcome these challenges include comprehensive strategies to achieve 100% smartphone penetration among villagers, emphasizing the importance of integrating all community members into the digital fold. This initiative aimed to improve the quality of public services and invigorate local communication, reinforcing the village's social fabric and economic vitality through enhanced digital connectivity.

At the beginning of this project, the public administration set up a smartphone consultation center at the health center in front of the Hidaka Village Hall. As we summarized and analyzed the inquiries from the residents, we could see several challenges the elderly faced using smart phones. Key challenges identified included the following:

High Costs: Smartphones are considerably more expensive than traditional cell phones, deterring many elderly residents from switching. Additionally, those living in mountainous areas require smartphones and investing in better connectivity solutions like Wi-Fi, adding to the financial burden.

Familiarity and Ease of Use: Many elderly villagers are unfamiliar with smartphones' functionalities, making the transition daunting. Efforts to simplify terminology and provide hands-on support have seen some success, but overall, the learning curve remains steep for many.

Perceived Lack of Necessity: Many elderly individuals do not feel a compelling need to switch to smartphones. They have managed their communications with existing tools and personal interactions and see no benefit in changing to more complex technology.

The application of Prochaska's Transtheoretical Model (TTM) (Prochaska & DiClemente, 1983) provides a structured analysis of how elderly residents in Hidaka Village progressed through different stages of behavioral change regarding smartphone adoption. This model identifies five stages: precontemplation, contemplation, preparation, action, and maintenance.

Precontemplation (Step 1): Many elderly residents initially did not consider using smartphones. Their reluctance was often due to misinformation, a need for more understanding about the benefits of technology, or a general resistance to change. These individuals did not attend informational meetings and were disengaged from discussions about smartphone usage.

Contemplation (Step 2) and Preparation (Step 3): Over the first two months, those who attended the meetings or visited the newly established smartphone consultation center began to move from contemplation to preparation. They gathered information and started to see the personal benefits of smartphones, such as enhanced communication with family and access to health management apps. Residents were making decisions about benefits and barriers within their own personal lives, as described in Becker's Health Belief Model (Becker, 1974).

Action (Step 4): Some residents, convinced of the advantages, decided to adopt smartphones. This stage involved purchasing the device, learning basic operations, and integrating it into their daily lives. The local administration facilitated this by setting up support systems like the consultation center, which played a crucial role in assisting the elderly through this transition.

Maintenance (Step 5): For those who had integrated smartphones into their lives, the focus shifted to maintaining usage and exploring more functions. Community support, ongoing training sessions, and positive peer and facilitator reinforcement helped sustain smartphone use and mitigate the risk of discontinuation.

Establishing a smartphone consultation center in the village has begun to alter elderly residents' perceptions and engagement with technology. The center reported a noticeable increase in inquiries about using smartphones, particularly regarding health apps and other functionalities that can enhance quality of life (Fig. 5.1). The consultation center has become a crucial resource in educating the elderly on the potential benefits of smartphones, gradually reducing resistance and increasing curiosity and usage.

Implementation Framework: From Theory to Practice

To operationalize digital integration as a Primary Health Care (PHC) intervention, clear role delineation and decision-making authority are essential. Table 5.1 presents a resident-led implementation framework adapted from the RACI model (Responsible, Accountable, Consulted, Informed), tailored for the Hidaka Village context.

This framework addresses three critical dimensions:

Resident Agency: Priority-setting and acceptability anchored in residents' voices, embodying the principle of "nothing about us without us"

Professional Accountability: Clinical safety (nursing) and statutory compliance (municipal administration) clearly assigned

Transparent Governance: All stakeholders understand their roles, enabling efficient coordination and conflict resolution

The framework is designed to be adaptable to other rural communities facing similar challenges of aging, depopulation, and digital divide. Nursing students and practitioners can use this table as a practical checklist when planning community-based digital health interventions. To operationalize a resident-led digital

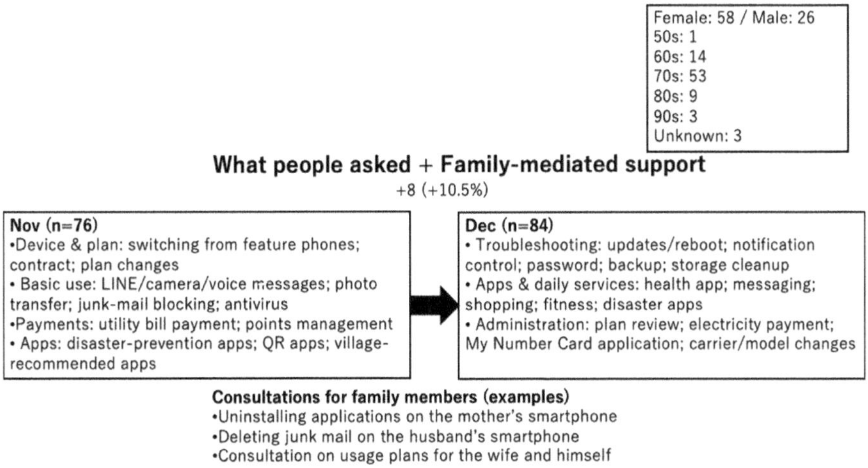

Fig. 5.1 Changes in consultations regarding smartphone use at the smartphone consultation center, Hidaka Village. (Source: Authors)

Table 5.1 Role sharing and decision-making across key implementation components (resident-led model)

Implementation component	Residents (older adults/caregivers)	Nursing professionals	Municipal administration	Technology provider	Final decision (accountable)
(1) Priority-setting and problem framing (health + DRR risks)	R/C	C	A (budget and mandate)	C	Residents (A for priorities) + Municipality (A for budget)
(2) Service and workflow design (apps, telemedicine, alerts)	C	A (clinical safety)	A (procurement)	R	Municipality (A), informed by residents' acceptability
(3) Digital literacy and peer support (training, consultation center)	A/R	R	C	C	Residents (A), supported by nurses (training quality)
(4) Data governance (consent, privacy, PHR sharing rules)	C	A	A (compliance)	R	Municipality (A), with residents' consent/acceptability
(5) DRR integration (warnings, evacuation support, continuity of care)	C	A (health continuity)	A (DRR planning)	R	Shared: Municipality (A for public plans) + Residents (A for household plans)
(6) Monitoring and evaluation (KPIs, feedback loops, policy adaptation)	C	A (evaluation design)	A (policy adaptation)	R (analytics)	Municipality (A), with residents' feedback as decision input

Note: *R* responsible (does the work), *A* accountable (final decision/answerable), *C* consulted, *I* informed. In practice, accountability may be shared: residents lead on priority-setting and acceptability, while the municipality remains accountable for public budgets and statutory compliance, and nurses for clinical safety

integration process as PHC, Table 5.1 summarizes the practical division of roles across key implementation components. In line with open governance, priority-setting and acceptability should be anchored in residents' voices, while clinical safety, statutory responsibilities, and technical quality are shared and clarified among stakeholders.

Key Insights From Table 5.1

Shared Accountability: In four out of six components, accountability is shared between residents and the municipality, reflecting the co-production nature of PHC

Nursing's Pivotal Role: Nurses are accountable for clinical safety, evaluation design, and health continuity—functions that bridge technical systems and human needs

Technology as Enabler, Not Driver: Technology providers remain in supporting roles (responsible or consulted), while human stakeholders retain decision authority

This resident-led model contrasts with top-down digital health initiatives that often fail due to poor adoption or sustainability issues. The framework ensures that technology serves people, not the reverse, aligning with WHO's people-centered care philosophy.

5.4 Case Study 2: Self-Care in Diabetic Patients and Integration of Disaster Preparedness

Implementing integrated people-centered health services requires a multifaceted approach that involves technological integration, stakeholder coordination, and community engagement. By aligning health services with the principles outlined in the WHO's global strategy, people-centered integrated care can create a more inclusive, effective, and responsive health system that serves the needs of its elderly population and contributes to the broader goal of achieving universal health coverage.

In defining service priorities based on life-course needs and preferences, a case study involving diabetic patients in Japan provides a compelling illustration. This population, particularly vulnerable during disasters, benefited from targeted disaster mitigation education that integrated health monitoring and community support (Nishigawa et al., 2016). This initiative, deeply rooted in holistic healthcare and technology integration principles, underscored the significance of personalized health services and community-based health planning.

As Tsuchiya notes, diabetic patients are high-risk individuals during disasters due to potential fluctuations in blood glucose levels triggered by stress and changes in living conditions, such as relocation to evacuation centers. Historically, during crises, these patients had deprioritized their chronic condition management due to more immediate survival concerns, leading to severe health complications (Tsuchiya, 2012). It is essential to empower patients to take control of their health through self-care practices tailored to disaster scenarios, including medication management, dietary adjustments, and emergency response actions. The project was conducted at the disaster-prone area, Kochi, Japan, with a high probability of experiencing a Nankai Trough earthquake. The purpose of this project was to examine the effectiveness of education methods for DRR for diabetics and the contents of the interactive education manual called "Disaster Notebook for Diabetics: Let's Prepare from Now." Before the project launched, Disaster Notebook was developed based on literature and existing disaster manuals. Then, a survey and interviews were conducted with certified nurses, specializing in diabetes nursing, to verify the effectiveness of Disaster Notebook, which was revised based on the interviews and feedback from the patients.

Outcomes and Impact

The program significantly improved patients' self-care competencies and disaster preparedness, reflected in:

Enhanced Self-Management: Patients reported better diabetes management during subsequent disasters, with fewer incidents of uncontrolled glucose levels.

Increased Engagement and Preparedness: The intervention increased engagement among participants, who reported feeling more prepared and capable of managing their condition independently during emergencies.

Increased Community Engagement: The program encouraged diabetic patients to engage more with their local health providers and community support networks, enhancing overall preparedness.

Policy Adaptation and Implementation: The program's success led to its recommendation for integration into the national disaster preparedness plans, with adaptations for other chronic conditions.

This case study underscores the importance of incorporating health technology and community-centric approaches to address the specific needs of vulnerable populations. By focusing on proactive education and preparedness, healthcare systems can significantly mitigate the impact of disasters on individuals with chronic diseases, aligning with broader goals of responsive and person-centered healthcare provision.

This case study highlights the critical role of tailored health interventions in enhancing disaster preparedness among high-risk groups. It exemplifies the effective use of health technology assessments in refining and optimizing health service delivery. The approach ensures that health services are continuously adapted to meet the dynamic needs of the population, thereby supporting the broader objectives of integrated, people-centered health services.

5.4.1 Generalizing the Diabetes–DRR Education Model: Conditions for Scaling to Other Chronic Diseases

The disaster mitigation education for diabetic patients (Nishigawa & Nojima, 2016; Tsuchiya, 2012) demonstrates how disease-specific needs can be systematically integrated into community-level DRR planning. This model is generalizable to other chronic conditions prevalent in aging rural communities (Table 5.2).

Core elements (cross-cutting):

- A minimum personal health record (PHR) that works in low-connectivity conditions (offline-first): diagnosis list, medication list, allergies, key baseline values, and care contacts.
- Medication and supply continuity plan: minimum stock levels, refill timing, and substitute options during disruption.

Table 5.2 Generalizing diabetes—DRR education models to scale other chronic diseases

Chronic condition	Key PHR elements	Disaster-specific risks	Required digital functions	Community support needs
Diabetes	Blood glucose logs, insulin dosage, carb counting	Medication/supply disruption, stress-induced hyperglycemia, foot injury risk in evacuation	Medication reminder, supply tracker, emergency contact list, glucose trend visualization	Peer support groups, medication stockpiling guidance, shelter meal planning
Heart failure	Daily weight, BP, fluid intake, symptom diary	Medication interruption, physical strain during evacuation, cold stress, salt intake at shelters	Weight/BP trend alerts, medication adherence tracker, exertion monitoring, emergency decompensation protocol	Home telemonitoring link, shelter environment modification, early warning system
COPD	Peak flow, inhaler use, symptom log, oxygen saturation	Inhaler/nebulizer disruption, home oxygen/power contingency, infection risk, poor air quality at shelters	Inhaler/nebulizer inventory, oxygen supply tracker, air quality alerts, infection prevention checklist	Alternate facility mapping, shelter ventilation standards, smoking cessation support
Dialysis	Dialysis schedule, vascular access status, fluid/ electrolyte balance, diet log	Alternate facility access, emergency renal diet, vascular access protection during transport	Dialysis center mapping (with disaster capacity), emergency diet calculator (K/P/ fluid), transport coordination	Transportation network, emergency dialysis protocol, caregiver training on access protection
Dementia	Medication adherence, daily routine checklist, wandering incidents, behavioral changes	Identification loss, wandering in unfamiliar shelters, routine disruption leading to delirium, caregiver stress	GPS tracking (opt-in), medication alarm, routine visualization (photo-based daily schedule), caregiver respite alert	Anti-wandering measures (ID bracelets, shelter layout), caregiver communication network, familiar object packing list

- Individualized evacuation and shelter plan: mobility needs, power needs (devices/oxygen), dietary requirements, and caregiver roles.
- Communication tree: family, neighbors, community leaders, and health providers; agreed check-in times and backup channels.
- Simple decision rules (red flags) and action cards: when to seek help, when to evacuate early, and where to go.

5.5 Conclusion

The World Health Organization's Global Strategy on Integrated People-Centered Health Services 2016–2026 advocates for health services that revolve around the preferences and needs of individuals, families, and communities. A case study involving diabetic patients in Japan demonstrates the critical importance of service priorities based on life-course needs and preferences. This particularly vulnerable population during disasters has benefited from targeted disaster mitigation education that integrates health technology and community support. Hidaka Village and similar communities can develop strong, equitable, and innovative health systems by embracing these recommendations. These systems can adapt to the rapid changes and challenges of the digital age, ultimately improving health outcomes and enhancing community quality of life. In the future, new technologies such as data algorithms, distributed autonomous organizations (DAOs), and non-fungible tokens (NFTs) will be utilized to manage and protect medical data effectively. These technologies can also streamline operations, increasing transparency and trust in the healthcare system. In addition to developing local human resources, creating an atmosphere that invites outside experts and investors who can bring in digital expertise is necessary. In light of these considerations, financial considerations are crucial. To this end, digital solution providers should consider the scalability and adaptability so that they can be applied in multiple regions. Digital solution providers must find stable funding sources, which can be a combination of direct and indirect funding, grants, and community investment.

Study Guide Questions

These questions are designed to help readers—whether you are a practicing APN at Level III, aspiring to this role, or supporting competency development in disaster nursing—apply concepts from this chapter to real-world practice. Each question aligns with specific ICN Disaster Nursing Core Competency domains and emphasizes digital health equity, rural community empowerment, and integrated people-centered health services in disaster contexts.

Questions

1. *Preparation and Planning*

   This chapter presents the conceptual pathway linking the digital divide to health inequity to increased disaster risk. Conduct a digital divide assessment in your community or organization, specifically examining elderly populations and rural residents. Using the WHO Global Strategy on Integrated People-Centered Health Services framework discussed in this chapter, develop a preparedness plan that addresses digital literacy, technology access, and social participation. How would you measure progress in reducing the digital divide and its impact on disaster resilience?

2. *Communication*

   Analyze the Hidaka Village case study, which demonstrates smartphone integration into elderly residents' daily routines and disaster preparedness. Design a technology-enabled communication and intervention strategy for your context that balances the benefits of digital tools with the limitations and preferences of vulnerable populations. How would you ensure that digital transformation enhances rather than replaces human connection and community social capital?
3. *Safety and Security*

   This chapter discusses how the digital divide can exacerbate vulnerabilities during disasters. What ethical considerations arise when implementing digital health technologies in communities with varying levels of digital literacy? How would you address issues of informed consent, data privacy, digital surveillance, and equitable access? Propose governance structures that protect vulnerable populations while enabling the benefits of digital transformation.
4. *Incident Management*

   Drawing from the diabetes self-care case study and the Future Recommendations for Integrated People-Centered Health Services (Table 5.2), design an implementation protocol for integrating chronic disease management with disaster preparedness in rural or underserved communities. How would you ensure continuity of care during disasters? What role would digital health tools play in both routine care and emergency response? How would recovery planning address the specific needs of people with chronic conditions?
5. *Community Engagement*

   This chapter emphasizes engagement and participation of elderly residents in designing health services. Reflect on the principles of Community-Based Participatory Research (CBPR) as they apply to digital health implementation. How would you facilitate genuine community ownership of digital health initiatives? What capacity-building strategies would prepare nurses at all levels to serve as facilitators of community-driven digital transformation rather than simply implementers of top-down technology solutions?
6. *Integration*

   This chapter discusses Japan's demographic challenges (population decline, aging, and depopulation of rural areas) and positions digital transformation as part of the solution. However, technology alone is insufficient. Synthesize the concepts presented in this chapter to propose a sustainable model for rural health systems that integrates digital tools, community social capital, inter-generational connections, and disaster resilience. How would you evaluate the success of such a model? What indicators would demonstrate both improved health outcomes and enhanced community well-being?

Acknowledgments The authors thank Seiko Iimura (research assistant, Kobe City College of Nursing) for her editorial assistance and reference management. Generative AI tools assisted with drafting and language refinement; all content was critically reviewed and approved by the authors. The authors express deep appreciation to the residents, community health workers, and local government partners in rural Kochi Prefectures who contributed their experiences and insights to this chapter. The work of Peace Winds Japan's disaster response teams is gratefully acknowledged.

Author Contributions Conceptualization: Yuri Machida, Megumi Fujii, Sakiko Kanbara. Field practice and case documentation: Yuri Machida, Megumi Fujii. Writing—original draft: Sakiko Kanbara; contributions from Yuri Machida and Megumi Fujii. Writing—review and editing: all authors; editorial and linguistic assistance provided by a research assistant (Seiko Iimura). Literature search and reference management: research assistant (Seiko Iimura). AI-assisted drafting: Generative AI tools were used to support structuring and language refinement under the supervision of Sakiko Kanbara.

References

Anderson, M., & Perrin, A. (2017). *Tech adoption climbs among older adults*. Pew Research Center. https://www.pewresearch.org/internet/2017/05/17/tech-adoption-climbs-among-older-adults/. Accessed 30 Apr 2025

Becker, M. H. (1974). The health belief model and sick role behavior. *Health Education Monographs., 2*(4), 409–419. https://doi.org/10.1177/109019817400200407

Cabinet Office. (2021). *Science, Technology and innovation basic plan* (Japanese). https://www8.cao.go.jp/cstp/kihonkeikaku/6honbun.pdf. Accessed 30 Apr 2025.

Cullen, R. (2001). Addressing the digital divide. *Online Information Review, 25*(5), 311–320. https://doi.org/10.1108/14684520110410517

Hidaka Village. (2021). *Hidaka village population vision revitalizing communities, people, and jobs*. Comprehensive Strategy. Available online: https://www.vill.hidaka.kochi.jp/kurashi/files/201732911312.pdf. (Japanese). Accessed 30 Apr 2025.

Kochi Prefecture. (2021). *Annual population estimates* (p. 14). Available online: https://www.pref.kochi.lg.jp/doc/t-suikei/file_contents/r02nenpou.pdf. Accessed 30 Apr 2025.

Laricchia, F. (2024). *Share of smartphone users in the United Kingdom 2012–2023, by Age*. https://www.statista.com/statistics/300402/smartphone-usage-in-the-uk-by-age/#statisticContainer. Accessed 30 Apr 2025.

Ministry of Economy, Trade and Industry. (2020). *Study Group report on Policies for Sustainable Regional Development*. (Japanese). Available online: https://www.meti.go.jp/shingikai/sme_chiiki/jizoku_kano/pdf/20200930_1.pdf. Accessed 30 Apr 2025.

Ministry of Internal Affairs and Communications. (2021). Part2. Chapter 4. Basic Data on ICT Field (White Paper). *Information and Communications in Japan*. Available on line: https://www.soumu.go.jp/main_sosiki/joho_tsusin/eng/whitepaper/2021/pdf/chapter-4.pdf#page=11. Accessed 30 Apr 2025.

Ministry of Internal Affairs and Communications, Japan. (2018). Part1. Chapter 4. Section 2. Current State of "Ties" through ICT (White Paper). *Information and Communications in Japan*. Available online: https://www.soumu.go.jp/johotsusintokei/whitepaper/eng/WP2018/chapter-4.pdf#page=2. Accessed 30 Apr 2025.

Ministry of Internal Affairs and Communications, Japan. (2022). *Telecommunication usage trend survey*. https://www.soumu.go.jp/johotsusintokei/tsusin_riyou/data/eng_tsusin_riyou02_2021.pdf. Accessed 30 Apr 2025.

Nishigawa, M., & Nojima, S. (2016). Disaster mitigation education for diabetics using disaster notebook for diabetics: Let's prepare from now. *Journal of Kochi Women's University Academy of Nursing., 42*(1).

Prochaska, J. O., & DiClemente, C. C. (1983). Stages and processes of self-change of smoking: Toward an integrative model of change. *Journal of Consulting and Clinical Psychology, 51*(3), 390–395.

Rad, J. (2025). Health inequities: A persistent global challenge from past to future. *International Journal for Equity in Health, 24*(1), 148.

Sarwar, M., & Soomro, T. R. (2013). Impact of smartphones on society. *European Journal of Scientific Research, 92*(2), 216–226.

Shaw, L. H., & Gant, L. M. (2002). In defense of the internet: the relationship between Internet communication and depression, loneliness, self-esteem, and perceived social support. *Cyberpsychology & Behavior, 5*(2), 157–171. https://doi.org/10.1089/109493102753770552. Accessed 30 Apr 2025.

The China Internet Network Information Center (CNNIC). (2021). *The 47th statistical report on China's internet development in 2020.* http://www.cac.gov.cn/2021-02/03/c_1613923422728645.htm. Accessed 30 Apr 2025.

The World Economic Forum. (2021). *The global risks report 2021 16th edition.* Available on line: https://www3.weforum.org/docs/WEF_The_Global_Risks_Report_2021.pdf. Accessed 30 Apr 2025.

Tsuchiya, Y. (2012). Proposals for diabetes countermeasures from the perspective of the earthquake I experienced. From the Great East Japan Earthquake. Iwate Prefecture 4. *Diabetes Frontier, 23*(2), 156–160. (Japanese).

World Health Organization. (2015). *WHO global strategy on people-centered and integrated health services: interim report.* Available online: https://iris.who.int/handle/10665/155002. Accessed 30 Apr 2025.

6 Gender, Diversity, and Digital Transformation in Disaster Risk Reduction: Methodological Leadership for Diversity, Equity, and Inclusion in Health Crisis Management

Sakiko Kanbara and Noriko Hatakeyama

6.1 Introduction: This Chapter as a DEI Methodological Leader

In an era of escalating climate risk, rapid demographic change, and widening social inequality, disaster risk reduction (DRR) and health crisis management can no longer be approached through a one-size-fits-all lens. What remains invisible in conventional plans—unpaid care work, informal support networks, and the structural vulnerabilities of marginalized groups—often determines who survives, who recovers, and who is left behind.

This chapter positions gender not as a narrow demographic variable but as a transformative entry point for understanding and addressing broader issues of diversity, equity, and inclusion (DEI) in disaster nursing and public health. Building on the community-based participatory action research (CBPR) foundations described in Chap. 5 and providing a methodological bridge toward the data-driven approaches elaborated in Chap. 7, this chapter demonstrates how DEI can be operationalized as a rigorous method rather than an abstract value. We integrate four methodological pillars. First, transformative gender mainstreaming (WHO, 2019) provides a theory of change that moves beyond awareness and sensitivity toward structural transformation. Second, digital transformation—conceptualized through Society 5.0 (Cabinet Office, 2015) and Kanbara's integration of the OODA loop, SOAP nursing records, and community diagnosis—shows how real-time decision support can be designed to advance equity rather than exacerbate divides (Kanbara et al., 2025).

S. Kanbara (✉)
Faculty of Nursing, Kobe City College of Nursing, Kobe, Japan
e-mail: s-kanbara@kobe-ccn.ac.jp

N. Hatakeyama
Faculty of Health Care and Nursing, Juntendo University, Tokyo, Japan
e-mail: n.hatakeyama.zo@juntendo.ac.jp

S. Kanbara (ed.), *Transformative Community Health Nursing*,
https://doi.org/10.1007/978-3-032-24405-5_6

Third, immersive cultural competency (XR-enabled empathy building) offers a way to make the invisible labor and lived realities of disasters experientially understandable, thereby strengthening reflective practice. Fourth, a multi-layered health system perspective (self-care → primary health care → public health) clarifies how local agency, mutual aid, and institutional support can be connected into a coherent resilience ecosystem. Together, these pillars form a practical framework for Jimoto–Sosei Kango (Community-Based Nursing for Local Resilience, a closer look in Chap. 7): a nursing paradigm in which care is not merely delivered to communities but co-created with communities, rooted in local knowledge and sustained through local governance and everyday practice.

This chapter is also intentionally aligned with global agendas: SDG 5 (gender equality) as a lens for SDG 3 (health and well-being), SDG 11 (sustainable cities and communities), and SDG 13 (climate action); the Sendai Framework's (UNDRR, 2015) emphasis on understanding disaster risk through participatory and people-centered approaches; and the WHO framework of Health Emergency and Disaster Risk Management (Health EDRM). By linking local practice with global standards, this chapter offers a model that is globally applicable yet locally adaptable.

6.2 Theoretical Framework—Transformative Gender Mainstreaming and Health Equity

6.2.1 From Gender Awareness to Structural Transformation

The WHO Handbook, Integrating Gender into the Curricula for Health Professionals (WHO, 2006) emphasizes that gender integration progresses through three levels: awareness (recognizing gender as a relevant variable), sensitivity (understanding that gender shapes differential health risks and experiences), and a transformative level (challenging and changing the power structures that produce inequities). In disaster contexts, awareness and sensitivity are necessary but insufficient. A transformative approach requires redesigning preparedness systems so that those most affected by risk—women, older adults, persons with disabilities, migrants, and other marginalized groups—are positioned as co-creators with real decision-making power. This is the methodological shift from "including women" toward rebuilding governance, knowledge production, and care systems to prevent exclusion. For Jimoto–Sosei Kango, this transformative orientation means that nursing practice extends beyond clinical care to include facilitation of community deliberation, recognition of structural vulnerability, and co-design of locally sustainable resilience practices.

6.2.2 Unpaid Care Work as a Critical Disaster Vulnerability

Unpaid care work refers to essential but often unrecognized activities that sustain life and health in daily living: childcare and eldercare, food preparation and nutrition management, hygiene and sanitation maintenance, basic primary health care and symptom monitoring, emotional and psychosocial support, and community cohesion activities.

Quantitatively, unpaid care work is a massive, gendered "invisible infrastructure." Based on time-use surveys in 64 countries, the International Labour Organization (ILO) estimates that 16.4 billion hours are spent in unpaid care work every day—equivalent to 2.0 billion people working 8 h per day without pay. Women perform 76.2% of the total hours and spend on average 3.2 times more time than men (4 h 25 m vs. 1 h 23 m per day). If valued at an hourly minimum wage, unpaid care work would amount to about 9% of global GDP (ILO, 2018).

In Japan, the 2021 Survey on Time Use and Leisure Activities reports that the average daily time spent in unpaid work is 1 h 19 min for men and 3 h 56 min for women, and there is a gap of 2 h 37 min (Statistics Bureau of Japan, 2022). This gender gap matters for disaster health management because the caregivers who already have constrained time budgets are also those most likely to be relied upon when evacuation, continuity of medication, hygiene, nutrition, and psychosocial support become urgent. During disasters, unpaid care work intensifies and becomes more complex—often under conditions of resource scarcity, disrupted infrastructure, overcrowded evacuation settings, and ongoing risk of disease outbreaks. Yet it frequently remains invisible to formal response systems, even though it directly shapes survival and recovery. Because care responsibilities are unequally distributed, unpaid care work is also a gendered and intersectional vulnerability. Many women and older caregivers shoulder a disproportionate burden, and people with limited mobility, chronic illness, or reduced access to information may depend on caregivers for evacuation and continuity of care.

This chapter, therefore, treats unpaid care work as a measurable and actionable analytic unit rather than a "soft" issue. Our research approach, developed through the Society 5.0 framework (Kanbara et al., 2022), positions technology not as a replacement for human care but as a tool for making invisible labor visible and supporting community-centered decision-making. Later sections operationalize this through complementary methods: (1) the OODA×SOAP-based participatory protocol (Sect. 6.4.1) integrates care work into structured data flows—making it visible as subjective narratives, objective observations, professional assessments, and actionable plans; and (2) XR-enabled immersive learning (Sect. 6.5.2) translates care realities into spatial, experiential scenarios where learners can enter disaster environments and understand care burdens through embodied perspective-taking. This dual approach—participatory data generation and immersive learning—provides an empirical pathway for translating the often abstract concept of unpaid care work into observable, teachable, and measurable components of disaster preparedness.

6.2.3 Social Determinants of Health in Crisis Contexts

Health equity in disasters requires distinguishing health inequalities (measurable differences in health outcomes) from health inequities (avoidable, unjust, and systematic differences). Disasters magnify inequities because they disrupt the conditions in which people live and care for one another.

Disaster-specific social determinants include: access to information (language barriers, digital divides, and trusted channels); physical environments (housing quality, neighborhood safety, and evacuation routes); social networks (bonding vs. bridging ties, social isolation, and gender segregation); economic resources (employment stability, savings, and insurance); and care responsibilities (family structure, disability, and chronic illness). A DEI-oriented disaster plan, therefore, cannot be limited to hazard maps and evacuation routes. It must also be a care plan: identifying who will need support, what kinds of support are feasible, and how everyday systems of mutual aid can be strengthened before a crisis.

6.2.4 Intersectionality: Beyond Single-Axis Analysis

Intersectionality highlights that vulnerability is rarely shaped by a single factor. Gender interacts with age, disability, socioeconomic status, ethnicity/culture, household structure, and geography to produce distinct risk profiles and different capacities for self-care and evacuation.

For example, young mothers may face evacuation barriers linked to childcare and mobility; older women caregivers may face chronic health issues and responsibility for spouses or grandchildren; women with disabilities may experience double discrimination; migrants may face language barriers and reduced access to trusted information; and rural or coastal settings may present unique challenges in transportation, communication, and shelter operations.

Pandy's comparative research agenda explicitly addresses intersectionality by examining diverse contexts—such as aging communities affected by floods and earthquakes in Japan, multicultural communities in urban areas, and post-earthquake recovery settings in South Asia (Pandy et al., 2022)—seeking methodological principles that are transferable while remaining sensitive to local cultural and socioeconomic realities.

6.3 Case Study—Kochi Women's Disaster Prevention Leader Project

6.3.1 Transformative CBPR in Action

The Kochi Women's Disaster Prevention Leader Project provides a concrete example of how a gender-transformative CBPR approach can be implemented as a community-based nursing methodology (Jimoto–Sosei Kango). The initiative emerged from Kochi City's post–Great East Japan Earthquake efforts to incorporate a "gender perspective" into disaster policy, including stepwise actions such as (i) committees of female municipal staff generating recommendations, (ii) the launch of a disaster-preparedness course at the Kochi Gender Equality Promotion Center, and

(iii) collaboration between the disaster management and gender equality sections to reflect these perspectives in manuals and practice (Cabinet Office, Gender Equality Bureau, 2020). Methodologically, the project design aligns with WHO's equity-oriented program review framework, Innov8 (WHO, 2016) and adapts it into local, competency-based learning that explicitly addresses the intersections of equity, gender, human rights, and the social determinants of health.

Rather than positioning residents as passive recipients of training, the authors established the program, which was organized as community-based participatory action research (CBPR): residents and municipal staff learned together, identified local vulnerabilities, and co-designed interventions through iterative workshops, field activities, and reflection cycles. Furthermore, course graduates formed an ongoing alumni network—Kochi Gensai Joshi-bu (Kochi Disaster Mitigation Women's Club)—which functions as a flexible "adult club" for sustained peer learning and community action (46 members, including inactive members) (Kochi Gensai Joshi-bu). This continuity mechanism is methodologically significant: it operationalizes transformative gender mainstreaming by shifting authority and knowledge production toward those whose care labor and lived experience are often excluded from formal planning. Importantly, the project connected disaster preparedness with community care ethics. Participants approached disaster prevention not as a separate technical domain, but as an extension of daily caregiving, neighborhood relationships, and health maintenance—the everyday foundation on which rapid crisis response depends. In practice, this meant translating abstract "preparedness" into care-centered routines that people can actually do (e.g., rolling stock, food preparation without infrastructure, sanitation and hygiene planning, and imagination-based scenario work) and then sharing these routines through community-facing events and educational materials.

6.3.2 Workshop Curriculum as a Competency Framework

The Kochi curriculum was designed as an applied learning sequence that gradually moved participants from foundational knowledge to co-creation and leadership. Across sessions, participants developed competencies in gender-sensitive communication, participatory assessment, inclusive facilitation, and cross-sectoral coordination. Concrete learning methods included the imagination/timeline tool for visualizing cascading risks in daily life, field-based risk walks and mapping, and hands-on preparedness practices (e.g., pack cooking, rolling stock, and sanitation) that connect disaster readiness to everyday care (Cabinet Office, 2017) The program's structure can be summarized in four phases: (1) Foundation building, in which participants learn core disaster concepts and reflect on gender and social determinants; (2) Co-creation, in which they conduct walking tours, mapping, scenario exercises, and interviews to identify hidden vulnerabilities; (3) Implementation, in which they develop and test tools such as risk communication materials and practice-based workshops (e.g., family-centered preparedness and cooking/sanitation drills); and (4) Sustainability, in which alumni networks and train-the-trainer approaches support continuity, diffusion to other districts, and collaboration with municipal systems. The full workshop schedule—serving as an example of an "Agora"-style participatory learning space where diverse actors repeatedly gather, deliberate, and co-produce knowledge—is provided in Annex at the end of this chapter so the readers can use it as a replicable protocol, "introduction → visualization → consensus → implementation" in line with the learning phase and the community's context.

6.3.3 Social Capital and Gender Networks

The Kochi case illustrates why social capital must be treated as an infrastructure of resilience. Social capital refers to resources embedded in social relationships—trust, reciprocity, shared norms, and networks that enable coordination. Women's everyday networks—such as school and childcare connections, caregiving and welfare ties, neighborhood activities, and community organizations—often function as rapid information routes and practical support systems in emergencies. Kochi Gensai Joshi-bu explicitly frames its mission as training local female leaders, disseminating preparedness information, and building a prefectural network for disaster prevention. In practice, this bridging function is visible in community events where residents, universities, and youth groups collaborate—for example, local exchange events that combined rolling-stock outreach with cooking drills involving residents and student volunteer teams. From the perspective of diversity management, strengthening social capital requires intentional design to avoid exclusivity. The Kochi program, therefore, emphasized collaboration with existing (often male-dominated) disaster prevention organizations, encouraging mutual learning rather than parallel, siloed activities.

6.3.4 Outcomes and Learning

The primary outcome of the Kochi project was leadership development. Participants who initially hesitated to speak in public settings gradually acquired facilitation and advocacy skills through repeated practice in inclusive workshops and community events. Tangible outputs strengthened this process: for instance, Kochi Gensai Joshi-bu produced practical educational materials such as the "KOCHI Minna no Gensai Handbook," which integrates hazard-map checking, the Meguroll imagination/timeline tool, rolling stock, pack cooking, and sanitation guidance for everyday preparedness (Kochi Gensai Joshi-bu, 2025). At the institutional level, the initiative functioned as a boundary-spanning mechanism: official case documentation notes that members participated in the process of creating a municipal supply distribution manual and contributed a women's supplies checklist as an appendix. The group also engaged directly with local governance forums, raising issues such as information accessibility for stockpiles, diversity considerations in shelters, and gender-based violence prevention. Methodologically, the Kochi curriculum offers a transferable model: a competency-oriented, gender-transformative CBPR approach grounded in daily care practices and sustained through an alumni network that keeps the “Agora” learning space alive beyond the course itself.

6.4 Digital Transformation for Human-Centered Health Crisis Management

The participatory workshops and community-based planning described in Sect. 6.3 successfully generated rich experiential knowledge: women identified care burdens, redesigned shelter layouts, and built social capital. However, a critical question remains: how can these localized insights be systematically captured, analyzed, and integrated into institutional governance systems that operate across multiple communities and time scales? This is where digital transformation (DX) becomes methodologically essential—not as a technological upgrade, but as a translational infrastructure. In conventional disaster management, DX is often framed as real-time data systems, AI coordination, or logistics optimization. Such interpretations risk reinforcing technocratic, top-down governance models that marginalize community knowledge.

In contrast, this chapter reconceptualizes DX as: (1) a tool for visibility—making invisible care work legible to institutional actors; (2) a mechanism for structural integration—connecting micro-knowledge to macro-policy; and (3) a bridge between everyday care and institutional design—translating narratives into actionable frameworks. In other words, DX does not replace care—it makes care governable. Women-centered DRR begins with lived experiences that are rarely documented in formal disaster manuals: food preparation under resource constraints, hygiene management in crowded shelters, emotional mediation among evacuees, medication monitoring for chronic conditions, and relational coordination across diverse needs. These practices are critical in preventing health deterioration and disaster-related deaths, yet they remain invisible to governance systems.

The OODA×SOAP integration and multi-layered health system (Sect. 6.4.1) provide operational frameworks for real-time care coordination. However, a methodological gap remains: how do we ensure that digital tools genuinely transform participatory practice rather than merely digitizing existing processes? The women's DRR activities described in Sect. 6.3 are grounded in lived experiences, relational knowledge, and everyday care practices. These insights are powerful but fragile—they remain local unless systematically captured, analyzed, and integrated into planning processes. Therefore, the next methodological step is not a shift away from community-based approaches, but rather an expansion of them into design-support tools.

This is where analytical frameworks such as PICRAT become relevant. Kimmon's PICRAT model (Kimmon et al., 2020) is not a technical model but a reflective tool that enables us to evaluate whether digital solutions amplify, in this case, women's lived knowledge or simply replicate conventional practices in digital form. In other words: Does technology function as an amplifier of women's experiential knowledge, or as its replacement? The following section introduces new aspects of the PICRAT model modified by the authors as a critical lens for assessing technology integration in disaster nursing management. DX contributes by: capturing dispersed micro-knowledge through structured observation protocols; structuring narratives into analyzable patterns (SOAP records, Sect. 6.4.1); identifying risk clusters before health collapse occurs (preventive logic); visualizing care gaps in shelter layouts (immersive simulation, Sect. 6.5); and enabling inclusive participation in design processes (PICRAT analysis, Sect. 6.4.4).

This shift from reactive to preventive governance is central to Jimoto–Sosei Kango. Traditional disaster governance responds to complaints, incidents, or measurable failures. Women-centered DRR, amplified through DX, shifts the logic to preventive design: mapping vulnerability chains (e.g., sanitation anxiety → dehydration → health decline), simulating spatial stress through immersive tools, and supporting iterative policy refinement. The integration of Women-Centered DRR and DX thus produces what we term a Preventive Care Governance Model: Care Narratives → Structural Mapping → Preventive Design → Governance Integration → Digital Amplification. With this framing, the following sections introduce specific methodological components—not as technological solutions but as systematic approaches to translating community knowledge into institutional practice.

6.4.1 Integrating the OODA Loop, SOAP Records, and Community Diagnosis

Digital transformation in disaster contexts is often framed as a technical upgrade. In this book, it is framed as a methodological redesign: technology becomes a tool for equity, participation, and rapid learning.

Kanbara's methodological innovation integrates three logics that are rarely combined in a single operational framework. Boyd's OODA loop (Observe–Orient–Decide–Act), originating in crisis management, offers a time-sensitive decision cycle (Chet, 2020). SOAP (Subjective–Objective–Assessment–Plan), originating in nursing records, provides a disciplined structure for interpreting narrative and measurable information (Kanbara et al., 2025). Community diagnosis, originating in public health, extends the unit of analysis from individuals to populations, focusing on risk factor identification, resource mapping, and targeted interventions.

When these three logics are integrated, the result is a multi-layered decision ecology in which subjective narratives (community voices, lived experiences, self-care logs) and objective indicators (administrative data, sensor data, GIS, real-time dashboards) are continuously translated into professional assessment and actionable plans. This supports both everyday health management and rapid crisis response. Conceptually, the integration can be summarized as: OBSERVE/Subjective → community narratives and lived experience; ORIENT/Objective → measurable and contextual data; DECIDE/Assessment → professional judgment supported by analytics;

ACT/Plan → individualized evacuation plans, community preparedness actions, and policy recommendations.

6.4.2 Real-Time Data Integration and Decision Support

Equity-focused decision support requires that data systems remain human-centered and privacy-preserving. A participatory digital infrastructure should integrate multiple sources: citizen input (photos, reports, self-care logs), sensor networks (environmental monitoring), administrative systems (evacuation center capacity, medical facility availability), and open data (weather, transportation, infrastructure). To prevent surveillance risks and protect marginalized groups, privacy-preserving architectures are essential. In Itamiya and Kanbara's digital health crisis management design, mechanisms such as anonymization pipelines, role-based access control, and privacy-aware data sharing are considered prerequisites—not optional features (Itamiya et al., 2022). Visualization and accessibility are also methodological choices. Multi-language dashboards, GIS-based resource mapping, real-time capacity monitoring, and context-aware risk communication tools can support rapid coordination while ensuring that information is usable by diverse groups, including those with disabilities or limited language proficiency. This section prepares the bridge to Chap. 7: once communities have established ethical, participatory data collection and interpretation mechanisms, they can generate high-quality data for longitudinal learning, evaluation, and policy advocacy.

6.4.3 Technology Integration for Transformative Learning: The PICRAT Framework

While Sects. 6.4.1 and 6.4.2 focused on digital tools for real-time crisis management (OODA×SOAP integration, data dashboards), technology also plays a critical role in education and capacity building. How can digital technologies support transformative learning for disaster nursing and DEI competencies? The PICRAT model (Kimmons et al., 2020) provides a systematic framework for understanding technology integration along two dimensions.

The PICRAT Model
The model classifies educational technology use along two axes:

PIC Axis (Student Engagement):
- *Passive (P)*: Learners receive information without active manipulation
- *Interactive (I)*: Learners interact with technology through responses or navigation
- *Creative (C)*: Learners use technology to generate artifacts, knowledge, or experiences

RAT Axis (Technology's Functional Role):

Replace (R): Technology substitutes traditional methods without functional change
Amplify (A): Technology enhances efficiency, reach, or effectiveness
Transform (T): Technology enables learning experiences previously impossible

The matrix resulting from these two axes provides a systematic framework for evaluating and designing educational technology use in disaster nursing (Fig. 6.1).

Application to DEI-Oriented Disaster Nursing
Traditional disaster nursing education relies heavily on Passive-Replace approaches: learners read case studies about vulnerable populations in written form. This approach can convey facts but struggles to build empathy, cultural competency, or understanding of lived experience. Our MetaNurse project (Kanbara et al., 2022) explicitly targets the Creative-Transform quadrant, which is shown in the upper right column of Fig. 6.1: learners actively create understanding through embodied experience in contexts that would otherwise be inaccessible (discussed deeply in Sect. 6.5.2). This alignment with transformative learning theory (Mezirow, 1991) supports the chapter's broader commitment to transformative gender mainstreaming: technology is not merely delivering content more efficiently, but fundamentally changing what learners can understand and how they develop professional identity.

Why Creative-Transform for DEI?
The Creative-Transform quadrant is particularly crucial for DEI competencies because: (1) Empathy requires embodied experience—reading statistics about care work burden differs fundamentally from experiencing the physical exhaustion, time

PIC (Student Engagement)	RAT (Technology's Functional Role) REPLACE(R)	AMPLIFY(A)	TRANSFORM (T)
CREATIVE (C)	Digital reports instead of paper	Create digital disaster plan with real data & sharing.	XR Immersive Experiences (MetaNurse): Design & simulate complex, multi-stakeholder disaster scenarios inaccessible in real life.
INTERACTIVE (I)	Clickable e-learning modules	Online quizzes & case studies.	AI-driven branching disaster simulations
PASSIVE (P)	PDF reading instead of books	High-quality video lectures	VR observation of rare disaster procedures

Fig. 6.1 PICRAT matrix applied to XR-based disaster nursing education: Creative-Transform quadrant for MetaNurse. (Adapted from Kimmons, R., Graham, C. R., & West, R. E. (2020). Used with permission)

pressure, and impossible choices; (2) Cultural competency requires authentic context—studying cultural differences differs from navigating unfamiliar social norms, environmental constraints, and resource limitations; (3) Transformative change requires productive disorientation—challenging implicit biases requires confronting one's assumptions in contexts that create discomfort. Therefore, the XR approach described in Sect. 6.5 is not simply "using new technology" but a theoretically grounded strategy for achieving learning outcomes essential for transformative practice in DEI and disaster nursing.

6.5 Visualizing the Invisible—XR and Cultural Competency for Transformative Practice

6.5.1 Why Visualization Matters in DEI-Oriented Disaster Nursing

Many of the most consequential determinants of disaster outcomes are not readily visible in formal plans: who performs care work, who is socially isolated, who lacks transportation, who cannot access information, and who faces stigma when seeking help. DEI-oriented practice requires methods that can surface these hidden realities without reducing them to stereotypes.

While OODA×SOAP provides structured data flows (Sect. 6.4.1) and PICRAT offers an analytical lens for technology integration (Sect. 6.4), both approaches rely on abstraction—maps, diagrams, and protocols. Yet, many stakeholders, including policymakers and institutional actors with limited field experience, struggle to imagine the lived conditions inside evacuation shelters: the lack of privacy, the burden of unpaid care work, and the cumulative stress of resource scarcity.

This is where immersive simulation tools such as extended reality (XR) become methodologically essential. XR was not adopted as a technological innovation for its own sake. Rather, it functions as a pedagogical device enabling participants to experience discomfort, privacy constraints, and spatial limitations from multiple perspectives—including elderly persons, caregivers, and women managing unpaid care work under crisis conditions. This experiential layer serves two critical functions: (1) empathy-driven design—participants viscerally understand why certain shelter layouts create care burdens, enabling more inclusive design decisions; and (2) preventive governance—by experiencing potential problems before they occur, stakeholders can implement preventive measures rather than reactive adjustments. In other words, XR translates the abstract concept of "invisible care work" into tangible, embodied knowledge that can inform institutional design. describes the MetaNurse project as a concrete implementation of this approach (Fig. 6.3).

Narrative-based and participatory approaches make these realities speakable, but they do not always make them felt. For professional education and community leadership development, experiential understanding can be decisive: it shapes not only knowledge but also empathy, ethical reasoning, and the willingness to share power.

6.5.2 XR-Enabled Immersive Learning for Empathy Building: The MetaNurse Project

Building on the PICRAT framework's Creative-Transform quadrant (Sect. 6.4.4), our MetaNurse project demonstrates how XR technologies enable fundamentally new forms of learning that complement CBPR. Unlike passive information delivery or interactive simulations, XR enables learners to create understanding through embodied experience in contexts that would otherwise be inaccessible. MetaNurse emerged from a collaboration between STYLY—a VR/AR/MR spatial layered platform chosen for accessibility and inclusivity—and EpiNurse—a global network of disaster health professionals from Nepal, the Philippines, Indonesia, Thailand, and Japan (EpiNurse, 2023). Unlike fear-based disaster simulations, the goal is not trauma exposure. The goal is cultural competency and reflective practice: learners experience ordinary routines under crisis constraints, then engage in facilitated dialogue and action planning. This design supports competency development in gender-sensitive communication, recognition of implicit bias, and facilitation of inclusive decision-making—competencies emphasized in global guidance for gender-responsive health professionals. XR tools also support hybrid forms of fieldwork. When physical access to affected areas is limited (e.g., due to distance, cost, or public health restrictions), immersive materials allow sustained "real × virtual" engagement while maintaining ethical safeguards and community consent.

Technology Platform: STYLY for Global Co-Creation
The project utilizes nurses without technical training to create XR scenes using a web-based Studio interface; experiences are viewable via web browser, mobile apps, Oculus Quest, HTC Vive, and other VR headsets; creators from different countries contribute scenes reflecting their cultural and disaster contexts; and field-based photos, 360° videos, and survivor narratives are integrated with community consent. This design embodies transformative gender mainstreaming: those with lived experience become knowledge creators, not merely subjects of study.

Example XR Environment: "Safe Place" Evacuation Shelter Experience
One flagship MetaNurse module, "Safe Place" (Fig. 6.2), represents a post-disaster evacuation site co-created by nurses from Japan, Nepal, and the Philippines. The immersive environment includes traditional shelter structures (Japanese school gymnasium, Nepali temporary housing, Philippine barangay hall) arranged in shared virtual space, enabling cross-cultural comparison; realistic density and noise levels with ambient audio (crying children, coughing elderly, generators); and resource constraints visualized through limited toilet facilities with wait-time indicators, cooking areas with insufficient equipment, and inadequate privacy partitions. Interactive decision points guide learners through morning allocation of limited breakfast rations, midday navigation of toilet queues when a child urgently needs the bathroom, and afternoon community meetings where learners must decide whether to raise concerns about childcare facilities. Embedded narratives include

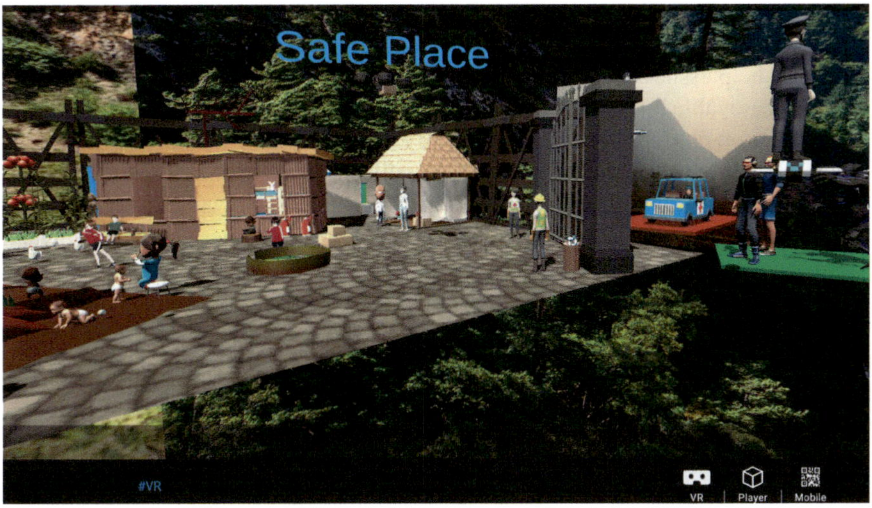

Fig. 6.2 VR "Safe Place": a digital agora for sharing diversity and care perspectives. (Created through STYLY)

visual indicators of invisible labor, such as care work time budgets showing water collection 3.8 h, meal preparation 3.8 h, and hygiene management 2.4 h.

This figure is a screenshot of the shared VR space labeled "Safe Place" (accessible via VR/PC/mobile). By placing elements essential for daily life and disaster response—such as housing, food, transportation, emergency medical care, and gathering spaces—within a single environment, it visualizes "invisible vulnerabilities" like care work, isolation, mobility challenges, and information access gaps. This allows participants to reference the same scenery while exploring concrete options. Within the integrated OODA×SOAP×CBPR methodology, it functions as a common foundation supporting Observe/Orient (Community Diagnosis + Interpretation through Gender/Intersectionality Perspectives). Following the reproducible procedures outlined in Annex, it connects to consensus building (Decide) and training/institutionalization (Act).

Evidence of Impact and Recognition

The practical value and innovation of this project have been highly recognized beyond academic circles. In early 2023, a joint project by Kanbara and Psychic VR Lab, titled "A Proposal for 'XR Disaster Prevention' Initiated by Citizens," was selected as a finalist in the "Weather as a Service Open Innovation Pitch 'Weather Up,'" a startup pitch contest hosted by the Japan Weather Association and featured on the economic media platform NewsPicks (NewsPicks, 2023). This proposal demonstrated a novel model that integrates the Japan Weather Association's highly accurate "Weather Data API" (Weather X) with XR platforms, superimposing potential virtual disaster scenes onto everyday spaces based on real-world weather data. Evaluations of this citizen-participatory approach have demonstrated a dramatic transformation in participants' engagement with disaster preparedness. Observations revealed a shift from conventional feelings of obligation ("I have to do this") and helplessness ("There is nothing I can do") to a positive, proactive attitude ("This is enjoyable," "This works for me"), facilitated through these immersive XR experiences on platforms such as STYLY. By experiencing virtual disaster scenarios linked to real weather data and engaging in collaborative sessions to identify "what I personally need," participants' individual lifestyles and values were directly reflected in their planning. Figure 6.3 are the examples of shelter variations in metaverse. This process successfully visualized diverse needs often overlooked in conventional, one-size-fits-all disaster planning—for example, a woman in her 50s prioritizing her favorite music and skincare sets during bad weather, or a man in his 30s seeking a balance of privacy and loose social connections in a long-term evacuation shelter. Ultimately, by elevating "what I designed for myself" into disaster-preparedness content that benefits the wider community, this approach substantiates the effectiveness of its inclusive core philosophy: a disaster-preparedness model that leaves no one behind because everyone can participate.

In this chapter, the metaverse-based visualization is positioned as an imagination and dialogue tool within the OODA×SOAP×CBPR methodology: it supports Observe (shared situational recognition of shelter conditions), Orient (gender-transformative and intersectional reflection on invisible vulnerabilities such as privacy, caregiving load, accessibility, and infection control), Decide (agreement on priorities and feasible resource allocation), and Act (implementation through workshops, drills, and institutionalization). The project exemplifies Jimoto–Sosei Kango's global–local dynamic: local knowledge contributes to a global platform, nurses

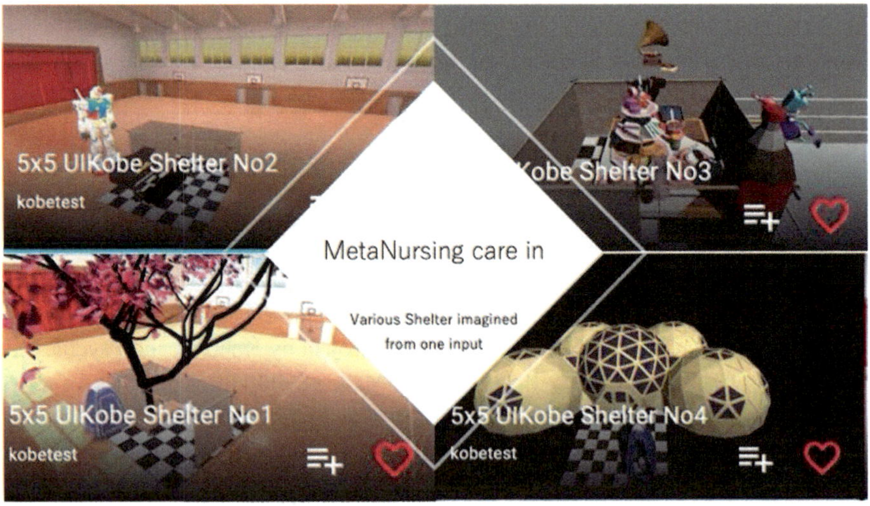

Fig. 6.3 MetaNursing "shelter variations" in the metaverse (STYLY): multiple evacuation shelter prototypes imagined from a single scenario input (NewsPicks production). Screenshot from the NewsPicks work "MetaNursing care in," presenting four alternative 5 × 5 "UIKobe Shelter" prototypes (Nos. 1–4) generated from one common input

support each other's capacity development across borders through shared XR environments, and technology enables rather than replaces human connection.

6.5.3 Cross-Cultural Competency and International Comparison

Disaster nursing requires not only local adaptation but also the capacity to translate learning across contexts. Cross-cultural comparison clarifies which vulnerabilities are structural and which are context-specific. Kanbara's broader international research program compares diverse settings (e.g., post-earthquake recovery and gender norms in South Asia, and other Asian contexts with different hazard profiles) (Kanbara et al., 2022). Such comparisons support a dual goal: extracting transferable methodological principles while respecting local cultural, socioeconomic, and governance differences. By embedding international comparison into both research and education—including XR-based learning materials—this chapter contributes to an evidence-informed, culturally competent approach that supports global knowledge exchange beyond 2030.

6.6 Implementation Protocol for Participatory Disaster Planning

This section translates the chapter's theoretical and digital frameworks into a practical protocol that communities and facilitators can implement. The protocol operationalizes Chap. 5 CBPR principles while generating structured observations and process data that can feed into the analytical approaches introduced in Chap. 7. The protocol also maps activities to WHO (2019) competencies for gender-responsive and equity-oriented practice.

Step 1: Recruitment and Team Formation

Objective: Establish a diverse, representative team that reflects community demographics and includes people who are often missing from disaster planning.

Key actions:

- Use multi-channel outreach through women's organizations, welfare associations, schools, workplaces, faith/cultural groups, and migrant support networks.
- Recruit across diversity dimensions (age, occupation, family structure, caregiving roles, disability inclusion, language) and clarify participation expectations.
- Form a gender-balanced facilitation/support team that can model inclusive practice.

WHO competencies emphasized: structural awareness (who is missing and why), inclusive communication, and ethical engagement.

Step 2: Safety Considerations and Ethical Safeguards

Objective: Ensure physical and psychological safety and protect participants' dignity and data rights.

- Obtain informed consent with clear explanations of data use, storage, and sharing; establish community oversight of sensitive information.
- Provide accessible venues (wheelchair access, childcare options, rest space, privacy) and flexible scheduling that accommodates care and work responsibilities.
- Use trauma-informed facilitation and codes of conduct to prevent harassment, discrimination, and power abuse.

WHO competencies emphasized: ethical practice, cultural sensitivity, and trauma-informed care.

Step 3: Facilitation and Capacity Building

Objective: Build the knowledge, skills, and confidence needed for diverse participants to contribute meaningfully and lead.

- Provide structured learning on local hazards, evacuation systems, gender and intersectionality, and the social determinants of health.
- Use participatory methods (walking tours, scenario role-play, mapping, affinity diagramming, interviews) to surface lived experience and local knowledge.
- Train facilitators to manage power dynamics, amplify quieter voices, and create shared ownership of outputs.

WHO competencies emphasized: gender-sensitive communication, recognition of implicit bias, and inclusive decision facilitation.

Step 4: Co-Creation of Plans and Tools

Objective: Co-design locally appropriate preparedness tools (plans, checklists, evacuation support protocols, communication strategies) that integrate diversity and care realities.

- Conduct community diagnosis to map hazards, population needs, and local resources; identify who requires evacuation support and under what conditions.
- Use the OODA×SOAP cycle to integrate narratives (subjective data), observations and records (objective data), shared assessment, and actionable plans.
- Pilot test tools through community events, school programs, and drills, then refine through reflection sessions.

Step 5: Digital Integration and Data Governance

Objective: Use digital tools to strengthen inclusion, coordination, and continuity of care while protecting rights.

- Develop simple digital interfaces for self-care records and family plans; ensure accessibility for older adults and people with disabilities.
- Create dashboards or shared resource maps that help communities coordinate support; design for multi-language communication and low-bandwidth environments.
- Establish participatory governance rules for data use: role-based access, transparency, consent, and safeguards against discrimination.

Step 6: Implementation, Reflection, and Scale-Up

Objective: Embed preparedness into daily life, sustain leadership, and connect community outputs to municipal and regional systems.

- Integrate preparedness activities into routine community care practices (health promotion events, welfare visits, school activities).
- Support peer mentorship chains among program graduates to sustain leadership and refresh participation across generations.
- Share outputs with municipal planning processes and open governance platforms so that community knowledge influences official plans.

The workshop curriculum summarized in the Annex offers a concrete example of how this protocol can be sequenced in practice as an agora-like process that moves from trust-building to action and dissemination.

6.7 International Comparison and Global Framework Alignment

6.7.1 Linking Local DEI Practice to Global Agendas

Diversity management in disasters is not only a local imperative; it is a global standard increasingly embedded in international frameworks. Positioning gender equality (SDG 5) as a methodological lens strengthens progress toward health (SDG 3), inclusive community resilience (SDG 11), and climate action (SDG 13).

The Sendai Framework emphasizes understanding disaster risk and strengthening governance through participatory, people-centered approaches. A gender-transformative CBPR design operationalizes this mandate by ensuring that risk is understood through the lived realities of those most affected and by building shared decision-making mechanisms that can persist beyond project cycles.

Similarly, the WHO framework of Health Emergency and Disaster Risk Management highlights the integration of health systems with DRR. By linking self-care, primary health care, and public health through participatory data and open governance, this chapter offers a nursing-led pathway for Health EDRM implementation.

6.7.2 Planetary Health, Society 5.0, and Equity-Focused Digital Governance

Planetary health perspectives underscore that climate change and environmental disruption are not external shocks but ongoing conditions reshaping health, livelihoods, and migration. DEI-oriented disaster nursing, therefore, requires long-term, adaptive governance rather than episodic response. Society 5.0 offers a vision of human-centered digital transformation. This chapter extends this vision to disaster and health crisis management, emphasizing that digital tools must be designed for equity: they should reduce barriers, amplify marginalized voices, and support transparent, accountable decision-making. However, digital transformation is never value-neutral. Ethical safeguards—including privacy-preserving data practices, accessibility by design, and participatory governance of data—are essential to prevent the reinforcement of inequality through surveillance, exclusion, or algorithmic bias.

6.7.3 Transferability and Contextual Adaptation

The framework presented in this chapter is intended to be transferable as a methodology rather than a single fixed program. Core principles—transformative inclusion, shared power, intersectional assessment, and iterative learning—can be applied in diverse contexts, from aging rural communities to rapidly urbanizing multicultural cities. Adaptation requires attention to local governance structures, cultural norms, gender relations, and resource constraints. This is why international comparison and XR-supported cultural competency are not add-ons but core methodological components: they help practitioners recognize both universal patterns of vulnerability and context-specific pathways to resilience. In practice, the question guiding adaptation should remain consistent with Jimoto–Sosei Kango: How can local people, using local knowledge and resources, co-create care systems that protect life and dignity before, during, and after a crisis?

6.8 Conclusion: Methodological Integration for Jimoto–Sosei Kango

This chapter has presented a methodological integration that treats diversity management as a rigorous practice of community-based nursing. By combining transformative gender mainstreaming, CBPR team building, and equity-focused digital transformation, the chapter provides a coherent approach to health crisis management that is both human-centered and evidence-generating. This chapter also

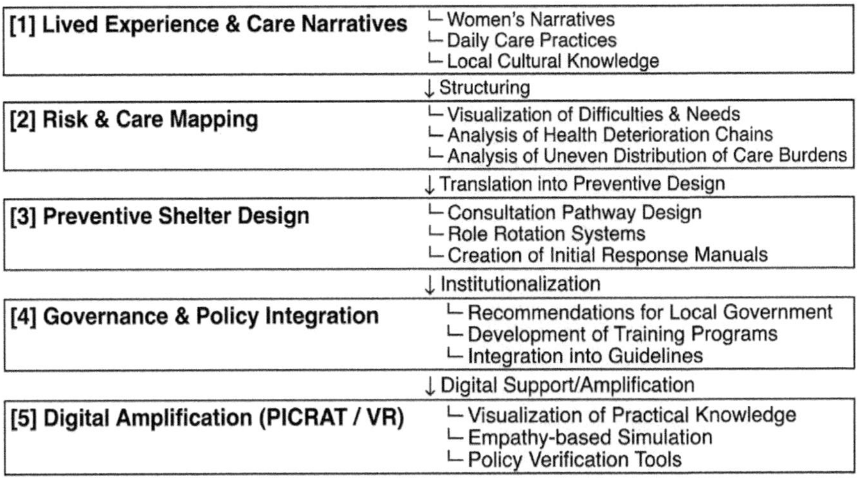

Fig. 6.4 Integrated process flow connecting lived experience to policy implementation. (Source: Authors)

clarifies a core claim of this book: Jimoto–Sosei Kango is not simply "community care," but a method for co-creating care locally—through inclusive governance, participatory knowledge production, and the activation of everyday care systems that sustain life during disruption.

This chapter has demonstrated a methodological progression that moves from lived experience to institutional design: Care Narratives (Sect. 6.3: Kochi workshops) → Structural Mapping (Sect. 6.4.1: OODA×SOAP data flows) → Preventive Design (Sect. 6.4: PICRAT evaluation + Sect. 6.5: XR simulation) → Governance Integration (Sect. 6.6: Implementation protocols) → Digital Amplification (Sects. 6.4.2 and 6.4.3: Real-time systems).

Figure 6.4 visualizes this integrated methodological progression. The framework demonstrates how women's lived experiences—particularly invisible care burdens—are systematically transformed into institutional policies through five interconnected stages. Each stage builds upon the previous, ensuring that community knowledge is not merely consulted but actively integrated into governance structures. This systematic translation process distinguishes Jimoto–Sosei Kango from conventional top-down disaster management approaches.

This framework illustrates the systematic transformation of qualitative, ground-level narratives—particularly regarding invisible care burdens—into structured data and analysis. This process translates micro-level insights into preventive designs, institutional policies, and digitally amplified solutions, bridging the gap between individual reality and governance. At each stage, technology serves not as a replacement for community knowledge but as a translational infrastructure that makes invisible care work visible and governable. This integrated model—what we term Preventive Care Governance—is particularly critical for super-aging, disaster-prone societies such as Japan, where conventional minimum humanitarian standards are insufficient.

The approach offers: (1) reduction of disaster-related deaths through early identification of care gaps; (2) health continuity in evacuation contexts through systematic monitoring; (3) institutionalization of lived care knowledge into planning systems; and (4) scalable preventive governance that adapts to local contexts. This model is transferable to other Asian contexts where community-based care cultures remain strong, as demonstrated by the Japan–Nepal comparison.

Kanbara's methodological contributions—integrating the OODA loop, SOAP nursing records, and community diagnosis—show how digital tools can support rapid decision-making without sacrificing equity, provided that ethical safeguards and participatory governance are embedded from the beginning (Kanbara et al., 2025). In parallel, XR-enabled educational approaches create new possibilities for cultural competency and empathy building, making invisible care labor visible and actionable. The Kochi case illustrates that when local people are trained and empowered as leaders, disaster preparedness becomes a living practice rather than a plan on paper. The project's curriculum, refined through iterative cycles of learning and reflection, demonstrates an "Agora"-style model of participation: repeated, open, co-creative gatherings in which residents, professionals, and institutions build trust, negotiate priorities, and generate actionable outputs. Finally, the program's learning design has been consolidated into the participatory workshop schedule presented in Annex. This schedule operationalizes the chapter's methodology as a transferable model—one that can be adapted to disaster-prone, aging, and socially diverse communities seeking to build resilience through locally created care.

Acknowledgments The authors thank Seiko Iimura (research assistant, Kobe City College of Nursing) for her editorial support and reference management. Generative AI tools assisted with drafting and language refinement; all content was critically reviewed and approved by the authors. The authors acknowledge the Kochi Gender Equality Center "Sole" and the Kochi Disaster Prevention Women's Network (Gensai Joshi-bu) for their pioneering work on gender-inclusive disaster risk reduction, and extend their gratitude to all community facilitators and participants whose contributions are reflected in this chapter.

Author Contributions Conceptualization: Sakiko Kanbara, Noriko Hatakeyama. Methodology and policy analysis: Noriko Hatakeyama, Sakiko Kanbara. Writing—original draft: Sakiko Kanbara; contributions from Noriko Hatakeyama. Writing—review and editing: Noriko Hatakeyama, Sakiko Kanbara; editorial and linguistic assistance provided by a research assistant (Seiko Iimura). Literature search and reference management: research assistant (Seiko Iimura). AI-assisted drafting: Generative AI tools were used to support structuring and language refinement under the supervision of Sakiko Kanbara.

Key Terms Defined

Transformative gender mainstreaming: An approach that goes beyond awareness of gender differences to actively challenge and change underlying power structures that create inequities (WHO, 2019).

Unpaid care work: Labor that maintains daily life and well-being but is not remunerated—including childcare, eldercare, housework, food preparation, health management, and emotional support—disproportionately performed by women and intensified during disasters.

OODA loop: A decision-making framework (Observe, Orient, Decide, Act) adapted for crisis and health emergency management to support rapid learning cycles and timely action. Originally from the Marine Corps, Boyd, J.R.

SOAP: A nursing assessment framework (Subjective, Objective, Assessment, Plan) integrating patient or community narrative with clinical and contextual data to guide care planning.

Community diagnosis: A public health method to assess population health status, needs, risks, and local resources, enabling targeted interventions and policy planning.

Jimoto–Sosei Kango: Community-Based Nursing for Local Resilience—a nursing paradigm emphasizing community autonomy, social collaboration, and sustainable local capacity building.

Social capital: Resources embedded in social networks, including information, trust, reciprocity, and collective action capacity (Bourdieu; Putnam).

Intersectionality: An analytical framework recognizing how multiple forms of inequality (gender, age, class, disability, ethnicity, etc.) intersect and compound.

Society 5.0: Japan's vision for a human-centered society integrating cyber and physical spaces through AI, IoT, and digital technologies for social good.

XR (extended reality/cross reality): An umbrella term for VR (virtual reality), AR (augmented reality), and MR (mixed reality) technologies enabling immersive and interactive experiences.

Annex: Participatory Workshop Schedule (Example of an "Agora" Model)

Annex summarizes the workshop-based curriculum that operationalizes the gender-transformative CBPR methodology described in this chapter. The schedule can be read as one example of an "Agora" approach: a recurring, open learning-and-deliberation space where residents, professionals, and municipal actors meet as co-learners, build trust, visualize risks and care needs, and co-produce action plans.

Session/Phase	Format	Core themes	Methods and activities	Expected outputs
Session 1: Orientation and Shared Baseline	Workshop (approx. 1 day)	Motivation, shared language of disaster risk, reflective entry into care and vulnerability	Self-introductions; shelter management simulation (HUG game); team presentations and debrief; mini-work on personal preparedness; "Meguro-ru" creation and discussion; participant presentations	Shared awareness of local disaster challenges; initial trust-building; personal preparedness commitments.
Session 2: Participatory Assessment and Gender Lens	Workshop + community fieldwork	Local hazard/resource identification; gender and inclusion in planning; linking to people requiring support	Walking/fieldwork to explore evacuation routes with local residents; identification of issues and barriers; map approach to synthesize findings; discussion of gender equality in disaster planning (guidelines); dialogue on disaster-vulnerable groups and referral/linkage mechanisms; reflection presentations	Community risk map drafts; articulated inclusion priorities; empathy for diverse evacuation and care needs

(continued)

Session/Phase	Format	Core themes	Methods and activities	Expected outputs
Session 3: Field Visit and Network Building	Site visit (2 nights/3 days) + reflection	Learning from affected communities; relationship-building; translating lessons into local context	Visits to disaster-affected areas; structured reflection workshop based on post-visit questionnaires; dialogue with local leaders and responders	Strengthened networks among participants and with external leaders; contextualized lessons for local adaptation
Session 4: Action Planning and Implementation Design	Workshop (approx. 1 day)	Applied skills for dissemination and district planning; practical care-oriented preparedness	Expert input (e.g., nutrition and meals in disasters); citizen-led examples (rolling stock, pack cooking, toilet issues); creation of group action plans; group presentations; feasibility review; disaster communication roundtable; program-wide reflection	Concrete action plans aligned with district disaster planning and shelter manuals; improved communication and facilitation skills
Ongoing: Community "Club" Activities (Alumni Network)	Continuous/ community-based	Sustainability, peer learning, mentoring, diffusion to districts	Information dissemination trials; local community workshops; peer consultation and presentations; collaboration with municipal and community partners; support for new cohorts	Sustained leadership pipeline and social capital; expansion of gender-and-inclusion perspectives in local DRR practice

Note: Session titles and activities are summarized from the original workshop plan. Local adaptation is encouraged (e.g., scheduling, facilitation methods, language accessibility, childcare, and disability accommodations) to ensure inclusion and safety

Study Guide Questions

These questions are designed to help readers—whether you are a practicing APN at Level III, aspiring to this role, or supporting competency development in disaster nursing—apply concepts from this chapter to real-world practice. This chapter serves as the methodological anchor for DEI across the volume. Each question integrates multiple ICN Disaster Nursing Core Competency domains and emphasizes transformative gender mainstreaming, intersectional analysis, CBPR methodologies, and digital tools for equity-focused disaster nursing.

Questions

1. *Transformative Gender Mainstreaming and Intersectional Analysis (Domains 1, 5, and 8)*:

   This chapter outlines a progression from gender blind → gender aware → gender-transformative practice, grounded in WHO frameworks. Critically analyze your current disaster preparedness and response systems using this lens. Where does your organization currently stand on this continuum? Beyond gender, how would you apply intersectional analysis (considering age, disability, socioeconomic status, ethnicity, and sexual orientation) to identify compounding vulnerabilities? Design a transformative intervention that addresses unpaid care work as a critical disaster vulnerability, as discussed in Sect. 6.2.2.
2. *Methodological Integration: OODA Loop, SOAP Records, and Community Diagnosis (Domains 2, 3, and 6)*:

   This chapter presents a novel integration of the OODA loop (Observe–Orient–Decide–Act), nursing SOAP records (Subjective–Objective–Assessment–Plan), and community diagnosis for human-centered health crisis management (Sect. 6.4.1). Apply this integrated framework to a specific disaster scenario in your context. How would you operationalize each component? How does this framework support real-time decision-making during crises? What are the advantages and limitations of this approach? How would you train nurses at different competency levels to use this framework effectively?
3. *Digital Transformation for Equity: XR, Visualization, and Cultural Competency (Domains 4, 5, and 6)*:

   Section 6.5 discusses extended reality (XR) and visualization technologies for making invisible vulnerabilities visible and building empathy and cultural competency. Evaluate the potential and risks of using immersive technologies (VR/AR) in disaster nursing education and practice. How would you design an XR-enabled learning module that develops cross-cultural competency and challenges unconscious biases? What ethical safeguards are necessary? How would you ensure that digital tools promote rather than undermine human dignity and therapeutic relationships?
4. *Participatory Action Research: The Kochi Women's Disaster Prevention Leader Project (Domains 1, 7, and 8)*:

   Analyze the Kochi Women's Disaster Prevention Leader Project case study (Sect. 6.3) as an exemplar of transformative CBPR in action. This project demonstrates community-driven workshop curricula, social capital building, and gender network development. Using the Implementation Protocol for Participatory Disaster Planning (Sect. 6.6), design a similar initiative for a marginalized community in your context. How would you navigate the six implementation steps (recruitment, safety/ethics, facilitation, co-creation, digital integration, reflection/scale-up)? What adaptations would be necessary for your cultural and organizational context?

5. *Global–Local Integration: Planetary Health, Society 5.0, and Digital Governance (Domains 3 and 8)*:
   This chapter links local DEI practice to global frameworks (SDGs, Sendai Framework, and WHO strategies) and introduces concepts of Planetary Health and Society 5.0 (Sect. 6.7). How would you translate global commitments to gender equity and inclusive disaster risk reduction into concrete organizational policies and practices? What governance structures would ensure that digital transformation serves equity rather than exacerbates existing inequities? Propose a framework for equity-focused digital governance that balances innovation with the protection of vulnerable populations.
6. *Professional Identity and Jimoto–Sosei Kango (All Domains—Integration)*:
   The conclusion positions this chapter as foundational to "JIMOTO-SOSEI KANGO" (community revitalization nursing). Reflect on your professional identity as an advanced practice nurse in disaster contexts. How do the methodologies presented in this chapter (transformative gender mainstreaming, CBPR, OODA–SOAP integration, XR visualization, and participatory protocols) collectively inform a new vision of disaster nursing leadership? Develop a personal professional development plan that integrates these methodologies into your practice. How would you mentor others in adopting this integrative, equity-focused approach?
7. *Synthesis Across Methods: DEI as Methodological Leadership (Cross-Cutting)*:
   This chapter explicitly serves as a methodological anchor for DEI across the entire volume. Create a conceptual map that shows how the methodologies presented in this chapter connect to and support the content of Chaps. 4 and 5 (and potentially other chapters). How does transformative gender mainstreaming inform multicultural community care (Chap. 4)? How do participatory methods support rural health empowerment (Chap. 5)? How does digital transformation for equity (this chapter) enable both transcultural nursing (Chap. 4) and age-inclusive technology adoption (Chap. 5)? This integrative question requires synthesis across multiple chapters and demonstrates Level III competency in systems thinking.

References

Cabinet Office. (2015). Society 5.0. (Concept note and policy communications).

Cabinet Office, Gender Equality Bureau, Government of Japan. (2017). *Collaboration with women trained in disaster courses to formulate disaster-related manuals* (Kochi City example) [PDF]. https://www.gender.go.jp/policy/saigai/program/pdf/jirei/12.pdf. Accessed 30 Apr 2025.

Cabinet Office, Gender Equality Bureau, Government of Japan. (2020). *Overview of the "Guidelines for disaster prevention and reconstruction from the perspective of gender equality"* [PDF]. https://www.gender.go.jp/english_contents/mge/drr/pdf/naikakuhu_BosaiGuideline.pdf
Chet, R. (2020). Boyd's OODA loops. *Necesse, 5*(1), 142–165.
EpiNurse. (2023). *MetaNurse project: Health Post for Everyone on Earth.* WIRED Common Ground Challenge. https://wired.jp/wired-common-ground-challenge/en/. Accessed 30 Apr 2025
International Labour Organization (ILO). (2018). *Care work and care jobs for the future of decent work.* International Labour Office.
Itamiya, T., Kanbara, S., & Yamaguchi, M. (2022). Chapter 8: XR and implications to DRR: Challenges and prospects. In S. Kanbara & R. Shaw (Eds.), *Society 5.0, digital transformation and disasters.* Springer.
Pandy, A., Kanbara, S., Pokharel, T., Sharma, C., & Shrestha, J. A. (2022). Chapter 22. Introduction to EpiNurse, emerging care, communication and health monitoring in Nepal. In S. Kanbara, S. Miyagawa, & H. Miyazaki (Eds.), *Disaster nursing, primary health care and communication in uncertainty.*
Kanbara, S., Hatakeyama, N., & Fukutomi, M. (2023). Trial of women's disaster prevention training that contributes to community disaster prevention plans – A study of social capital with Kochi Gensai Jyoshibu. *Journal of the Regional Disaster Prevention Plan, 26.* (Japanese).
Kanbara, S., Ozaki, Y., Oshima, M., Ando, T., & Rajib, S. (2025). *Integrated OODA-SOAP framework for citizen-centered disaster health management.* https://researchmap.jp/sakikokanbara/misc/52227650. Accessed 30 Apr 2025.
Kimmons, R., Graham, C. R., & West, R. E. (2020). The PICRAT model for technology integration in teacher preparation. *Contemporary Issues in Technology and Teacher Education, 20*(1), 176–198.
Kochi Disaster Mitigation Women's Club (Kochi Gensai Joshi-bu). (2023). *Disaster reduction handbook for everyone.* https://gensaijyoshi.jimdofree.com/kochi%E3%81%BF%E3%82%93%E3%81%AA%E3%81%AE%E6%B8%9B%E7%81%BD%E3%83%8F%E3%83%B3%E3%83%89%E3%83%96%E3%83%83%E3%82%AF/. Accessed 30 Apr 2025.
Kochi Gensai Jyoshibu: About. (Japanese) https://gensaijyoshi.jimdofree.com/%E3%81%93%E3%81%86%E3%81%A1%E6%B8%9B%E7%81%BD%E5%A5%B3%E5%AD%90%E9%83%A8%E3%81%AB%E3%81%A4%E3%81%84%E3%81%A6/. Accessed 30 Apr 2025.
Mezirow, J. (1991). *Transformative dimensions of adult learning*. Jossey-Bass.
NewsPicks. (2023). *Weather as a service open innovation pitch 'Weather Up'.* https://newspicks.com/movie-series/10/?movieId=2520. Accessed 30 Apr 2025.
United Nations Office for Disaster Risk Reduction (UNDRR). (2015). *Sendai framework for disaster risk reduction 2015–2030.*
Weather X. *Japan Weather Association.* https://weather-jwa.jp/en/. Accessed 30 Apr 2025.
World Health Organization. (2006). *Integrating gender into the curricula for health professionals: Handbook.*
World Health Organization. (2016). *Innov8 approach for reviewing national health programmes to leave no one behind: Technical Handbook.*
World Health Organization. (2019). *Health emergency and disaster risk management framework.*

Data-Driven Empowerment in Community Health (Kurashiki): The Mabi Care Map as a JIMOTO-Based Case of Open Governance

7

Sakiko Kanbara

7.1 Introduction: From Disaster Response to Data-Driven Resilience

Chapters 4, 5 and 6 have illustrated community-based innovation largely through projects rooted in Kochi Prefecture, where disaster risk reduction, digital inclusion, and inclusive leadership were developed as place-based practices. This chapter shifts the lens to a different kind of locality: the author's own *Jimoto* (home community), Mabi District in Kurashiki City, which was devastated by the 2018 Western Japan Floods. The author happened to be in Mabi from the day before the disaster and, while her home avoided inundation, she engaged in intermittent disaster nursing activities and community coordination on the ground. This positionality—being both a nursing professional and a member of the affected locality—clarifies why data-driven approaches matter: they are not "technologies applied to communities," but tools that help communities act with ownership (a sense of ownership) in conditions of uncertainty.

In other words, the core question of this chapter is not only how open data or mapping can support primary health care. It is how a community, through civic participation and trustworthy information practices, can convert shock into learning and recovery into long-term capacity—so that resilience becomes a shared, renewable asset of *Jimoto*.

S. Kanbara (✉)
Faculty of Nursing, Kobe City College of Nursing, Kobe, Japan
e-mail: s-kanbara@kobe-ccn.ac.jp

S. Kanbara (ed.), *Transformative Community Health Nursing*,
https://doi.org/10.1007/978-3-032-24405-5_7

Connecting to the Book's Core Framework: "Know Your Enemy, Know Yourself"

This chapter advances the book's central framework, articulated throughout previous chapters: "knowing the enemy" (understanding the hazard) must be paired with "knowing yourself" (understanding the community's characteristics, capacities, and constraints). In disaster contexts, this dual knowledge forms the foundation of actionable preparedness and response. Yet, as the Mabi case demonstrates, knowledge alone—whether codified in hazard maps, evacuation plans, or disaster preparedness manuals—does not automatically translate into protective action or equitable outcomes.

The transformation of knowledge into "actionable knowing" requires two parallel processes:

1. Data ecosystems that bridge formal and informal knowledge: Open data (such as the Mabi Care Map's geospatial information on functioning services, accessible shelters, and hazard zones) must integrate with Personal Health Records (PHRs) (such as the Imakara/Korekara Logbook's individualized medication, condition, and support network documentation mentioned in Sect. 7.4). Neither is sufficient alone. Open data reveals collective needs and resource gaps; PHRs capture individual vulnerabilities that are invisible to aggregate systems.
2. Trusted intermediaries and participatory governance: Technical information systems require human infrastructure—places (like Kanbara Gofukuten, the kimono shop that became an information hub), people (disaster nurses, community volunteers, local leaders), and protocols (such as the hotel evacuation pilot's attempt to preemptively coordinate private accommodation). These intermediaries do not simply "deliver" data; they co-create it, validate it, and translate it into context-appropriate forms that diverse populations can use.

This chapter's role in this book is to demonstrate how data-driven empowerment works (and sometimes fails) across four interconnected domains: situational awareness (do residents know what is happening and where to go?), decision capacity (can individuals and families make informed choices under pressure?), care continuity (are health needs tracked and addressed longitudinally?), and governance transformation (do power dynamics shift to enable community agency?). Each initiative examined here—the Mabi Care Map, Kanbara Gofukuten as an information commons, the Imakara/Korekara Logbook system, and the Kochi hotel evacuation pilot—contributes differently to these outcomes, revealing both the potential and the persistent barriers of data-driven approaches in disaster contexts.

By this chapter's conclusion, we arrive at an essential insight for Chap. 8: resilience is not built by data systems alone, but by the social infrastructure that generates, curates, and activates data as a collective resource. This realization sets the stage for examining governance structures, Community-Based Participatory Research (CBPR) methodologies, and the emerging role of "Society 5.0 Nightingales" who can navigate between technical systems, community knowledge, and policy influence.

7.2 The Kanbara Gofukuten Story: A Grassroots Community Hub

Although the Mabi Care Map was developed in the acute phase of the flood response, this chapter begins with Kanbara Gofukuten as an agora to foreground the trusted social infrastructure through which data becomes actionable care.

Beyond the digital mapping efforts, localized grassroots initiatives also played a vital role in sustaining the community during the critical post-flood weeks. One particularly notable example was the transformation of Kanbara Gofukuten—a traditional kimono shop operated by the father of a disaster nursing specialist (author)—into a multifunctional community support hub.

Situated within walking distance from affected neighborhoods, the store quickly became a physical anchor for informal relief coordination. Between July 11 and August 6, 2018, more than 140 residents and 147 volunteer supporters engaged with the facility, building trust through place-based mutual aid. Over the course of a month, the space provided:

- Well water to neighbors when the municipal supply failed
- Emergency communication and coordination point
- Child care so parents could focus on cleanup operations
- Volunteer lodging and meals for supporters from near and far
- Relief supply distribution to affected residents

These physical and relational networks of care complemented the Mabi Care Map's digital infrastructure. Information gathered at the shop—about which households needed assistance, who had health concerns, or where food was running low—fed into the participatory mapping process, creating an integrated flow between lived experience and open data.

This synergistic model revealed the power of combining technology with social familiarity: data became more meaningful when rooted in trusted spaces, and care became more effective when guided by real-time spatial intelligence. The Kanbara shop thus exemplified a form of embedded resilience, where intergenerational trust and adaptive use of everyday infrastructure empowered citizens to act during a crisis.

Reconceptualizing Kanbara Gofukuten: The Data Intake Point

Beyond its role as a relief hub, Kanbara Gofukuten functioned as "the data intake point" in Mabi's disaster response ecosystem—a critical but often invisible function in data-driven governance.

In formal disaster response systems, data collection typically begins with structured surveys, official damage assessments, or government agency reports. However, these top-down data streams often lag behind ground reality, miss nuanced local needs, and fail to capture the experiences of marginalized populations. Kanbara Gofukuten solved this problem by serving as a trusted space, where unstructured, "pre-categorized" information naturally accumulated (Fig. 7.1):

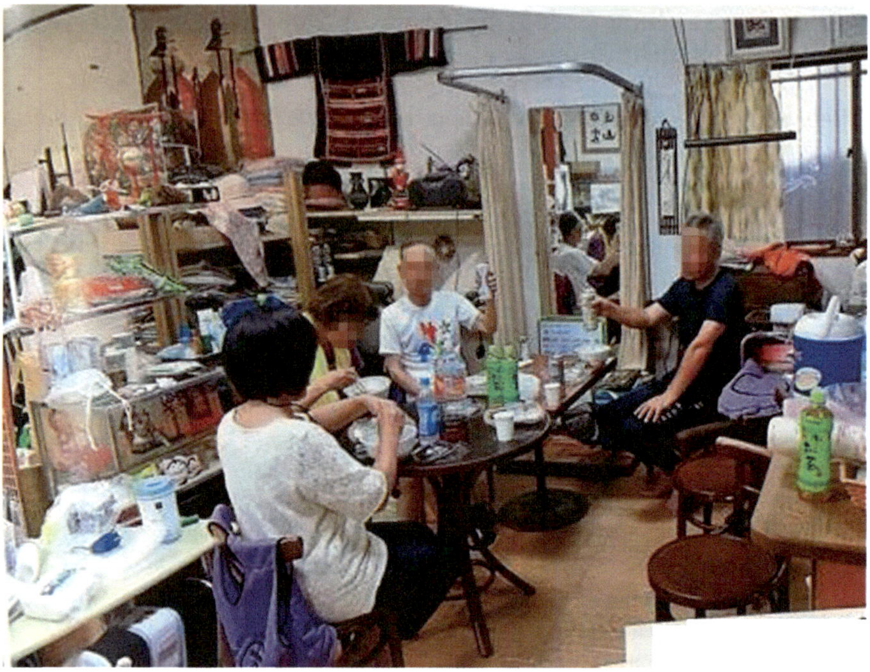

Fig. 7.1 Kanbara Gofukuten

- Observational data: Volunteers and residents conversing in the shop spontaneously shared information about which neighborhoods remained inaccessible, which elderly residents had not been seen, or which families were struggling with specific challenges (e.g., lack of baby formula, medication shortages, mental health crises).
- Need articulation before formalization: Residents could voice needs in their own language and context before those needs were forced into predefined categories (e.g., "I'm worried about my neighbor's mother who has dementia" rather than "elderly with cognitive impairment requiring evacuation assistance"). This preserved the richness and specificity that formal intake forms often lose.
- Trust-mediated data sharing: Because the shop was run by a community member (the author, a disaster nurse who grew up in Mabi), residents were willing to share sensitive information—health conditions, family conflicts, financial struggles—that they would not have disclosed to external aid organizations or government officials.

This "grassroots data generation" was then fed into the Mabi Care Map's structured geospatial database: locations of vulnerable individuals were mapped, service gaps were identified, and volunteer deployment was coordinated based on ground-truth intelligence. The shop thus served as a data translation layer—converting lived experience into actionable, shareable information without stripping away context or voice.

7.3 Situational Analysis: Mabi Case Study Through the Health EDRM Framework

This section analyzes the Mabi disaster using the World Health Organization's Health Emergency and Disaster Risk Management (Health EDRM) framework. From a nursing perspective, this case study examines the interplay between environmental hazards, social vulnerabilities, and the systemic collapse of primary health care (PHC) infrastructure.

7.3.1 Hazard and Exposure: Geographic Vulnerability

Geographic Context Mabi, a semi-rural district of approximately 20,631 residents (December 2024), sits at the topographically vulnerable confluence of the Takahashi and Oda Rivers on low-lying land reclaimed from floodplains. Importantly for this book's theme of locally rooted transformation, Mabi is the author's *jimoto* (hometown). The author happened to return home the day before the floods and, although her home avoided inundation, engaged in disaster nursing activities and community coordination throughout the crisis.

Historical Hazard Profile The Takahashi River basin has experienced major floods in 1893, 1976, and 1998. However, a 42-year gap (1976–2018) eroded institutional memory—newer residents who moved for affordability and proximity to Okayama City were largely unaware of this history. Ironically, Okayama Prefecture's reputation as the "Land of Sunshine" (lowest rainfall in Japan per JMA data 1981–2010) (JMA, 2020) fostered normalcy bias, where residents underestimated flood risk despite hydrological reality.

7.3.2 Social Vulnerability: Demographic and Structural Risk

Aging Population: Pre-disaster aging rate exceeded 30%. Many elderly residents lived in pre-1981 wooden structures or single-story homes without vertical evacuation capacity.

The Bedroom Community Paradox: Mabi's transformation following its 2005 merger with Kurashiki City created critical vulnerabilities: (1) absentee capacity as working-age adults commuted to Kurashiki and Okayama during weekdays, and (2) concentrated critical infrastructure—supermarkets, medical clinics, pharmacies, and schools built in convenient low-lying areas, ensuring simultaneous failure during flooding (Das, 2019).

7.3.3 The Crisis Event: Simultaneous Systems Collapse

Pre-Disaster Warnings (July 5–6) A stationary front had saturated the ground since late June. On July 5, Japan Meteorological Agency (JMA) issued Heavy Rain Warnings. By July 6, 10:00 PM, JMA upgraded to Heavy Rain Emergency Warnings (the highest alert level), but critically late—rivers were already overflowing and darkness had fallen. Kurashiki City issued an Evacuation Advisory at 9:50 PM, then an Evacuation Order at 11:16 PM, but many residents were asleep, lacked smartphones, or dismissed warnings due to normalcy bias (Kurashiki City, 2019).

The Night of Catastrophe (July 6–7) Between midnight and 2:00 AM on July 7, the Oda River's embankments collapsed in eight locations. Within 2–3 h, approximately 1200 hectares (one-third of Mabi) were submerged, with water levels reaching up to 5 m in some areas, completely engulfing single-story homes. Over 10,000 residents lived in the inundation zone. Emergency services received over 3000 rescue requests within 24 h but faced severe constraints: roads were impassable, helicopters were initially grounded, and first responders themselves required rescue.

Family Separation and Information Vacuum Evacuation patterns were chaotic and dispersed—relatives' homes in neighboring towns, car camping on high ground, and shrines and hillside facilities. Families were separated for 3–5 days with no communication as phone batteries died, power outages spread, and cell towers were damaged. The psychological toll of this uncertainty was immense. Adding to the trauma, reports of looting and theft by outsiders entering the disaster zone created fear and prompted some evacuees to risk returning to protect their property.

Infrastructure Collapse By July 7, critical infrastructure had failed comprehensively: 4600 homes flooded (1200 with above floor level inundation), 6000 households without electricity, the entire town without running water, 18 major routes blocked, and telecommunications severely compromised.

Shelter Crisis Mabi's three school gymnasiums (official capacity: 480) were overwhelmed by over 2000 evacuees by July 7 morning—more than four times capacity. Conditions deteriorated rapidly: insufficient toilets, poor ventilation, extreme heat (37 °C/98.6 °F), and overcrowding. Vulnerable groups (visually impaired, persons with dementia, pregnant women) received priority classroom space, but many families with pets or children with disabilities avoided shelters entirely, fearing stigma or inability to manage needs in chaos. Interviews with 15 mothers of children with intellectual disabilities revealed that they evacuated to relatives' homes instead (Kanbara et al., 2019).

Compound Health Hazards The disaster created overlapping crises:

1. *Heat-related illness and infectious disease*: Overcrowded, poorly ventilated shelters with compromised sanitation (sewage-contaminated floodwater).
2. *Chronic disease disruption*: Flooded Mabi Health Center, clinics, and pharmacies created medication shortages (insulin, hypertension drugs), and lost medical records.
3. *Mental health crisis*: Trauma from near-death experiences, family separation, and uncertainty triggered acute stress and insomnia.
4. *Nutritional deficiencies*: Carbohydrate-heavy food aid (bread, rice balls, curry served three times in 1 day per social media posts).
5. *Physical exhaustion*: Cleanup work led to dehydration, stress fractures, and musculoskeletal injuries.
6. *Caregiver burnout*: Survey data months later revealed *30% of respondents still "lacked energy to cook"* despite repairs, indicating profound mental exhaustion.

Temporal Pressure Seven of nine schools serving as shelters faced a mid-August deadline to reopen for the second semester, forcing a rapid transition from emergency to recovery phase (Miyamoto et al., 2023).

7.3.4 The Human Toll: Mortality and Invisible Burdens

Fifty-One Lives Lost 90% died by drowning; average age 73.8 years; 60% lived alone or with one other elderly family member; 70% found in their homes. Over 2300 residents required emergency rescue from rooftops by helicopter or boat (Das, 2019).

Unpaid Informal Care The disaster exposed the critical, often invisible, role of informal caregiving—disproportionately performed by women—including assisting elderly parents, managing children, and brokering information. The "daytime evacuation" pattern (leaving shelters during day, returning at night) made needs assessment challenging, as formal counts drastically underestimated actual needs.

7.3.5 The Capacity Gap: Hazard Map Paradox and Structural Failure

In March 2016, Kurashiki City distributed accurate hazard maps predicting flood extent. Yet, 51 died, over 2300 required rescue, and 4600 homes flooded. The system failed due to:

1. *Temporal paradox*: Maps arrived after high-risk zones were densely populated (post-2005 suburban development), too late for land use decisions, too early to trigger immediate behavioral change (1-in-1000-year event perceived as distant abstraction).

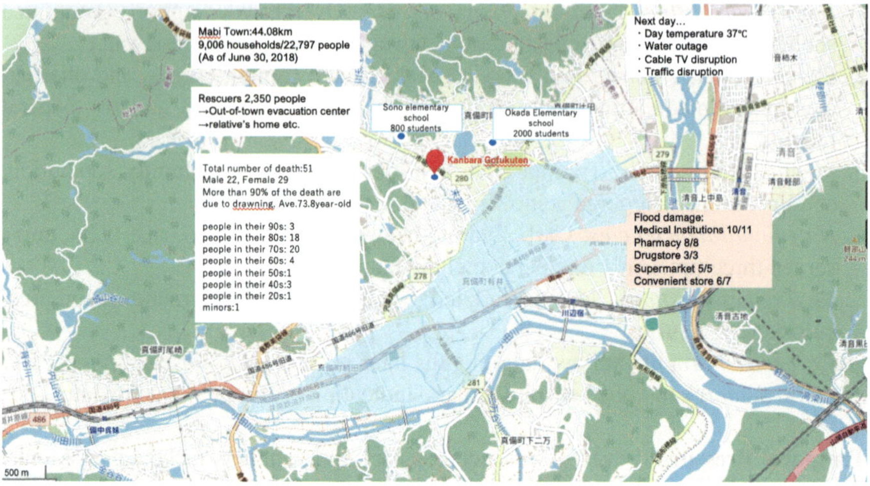

Fig. 7.2 Damage map (July 8, 2018, by author)

2. *Cognitive barriers*: Maps lacked actionable protocols—no regular flood drills (unlike earthquake/tsunami drills), ambiguous evacuation triggers, and no community-level social norms around flood response.
3. *Spatial vulnerability*: GIS analysis revealed 12 of 22 designated shelters (54.55%) were in the flood inundation zone (Sritart et al., 2020). When floods struck, the remaining accessible capacity was 1340 people (43.86% of the original 3110 capacity), with demand-capacity mismatches exceeding 600% at some shelters. Overall, 68 population points were completely isolated.

This "vulnerability of vulnerability" phenomenon—pre-existing structural weaknesses catastrophically amplified by disaster—demonstrates that data and technology alone cannot ensure resilience without addressing spatial planning, behavioral preparedness, and institutional coordination (Fig. 7.2).

7.3.6 Nursing Perspective: The Ethics of Being Present

The author's positionality—a disaster nursing specialist who happened to be home in her *jimoto*—created unique contributions:

1. *Immediate mobilization*: Coordinating informal relief within hours using local knowledge and relationships.
2. *Cultural fluency*: Understanding local dialect, social networks, and unspoken norms facilitated trust-building.
3. *Long-term commitment*: Unlike external aid that withdraws, being from Mabi meant enduring a stake in recovery.
4. *Ethical accountability*: Decisions made knowing she would remain part of this community.

This *jimoto-embedded coordination* bridged the gap between official data and lived reality, revealing invisible needs: families with disabled children avoiding shelters, elderly residents isolated in hillside communities, and non-Japanese speakers lacking accessible information (Kanbara et al., 2019). Disaster nursing requires situational interpretation grounded in trust—chaos contains patterns which, when mapped, can inform community-driven resilience.

7.4 The Imakara/Korekara Logbook: Analog PHR for Disaster Self-Care

Another complementary innovation to emerge during the recovery from the Mabi disaster was the use of the "Imakara Logbook" ("From Now Handbook") (Fig. 7.3) and later the "Korekara Logbook" ("Going Forward Handbook")—community-distributed personal health journals designed to support self-care and continuity of information in disaster-affected populations.

7.4.1 Origins and Conceptual Framework

Originally inspired by Japan's Maternal and Child Health Handbook model, these logbooks enabled residents to track their medical conditions, medications, key contacts, and emotional reflections across phases of evacuation and rebuilding (Miyamoto et al., 2023). The Maternal and Child Health Handbook has been a cornerstone of Japanese preventive health since 1948, providing a unified record that families maintain across different healthcare providers and life stages (Nakamura, 2015). The logbook concept adapted this proven model for disaster contexts, where medical records are often lost and healthcare access is disrupted.

The logbooks contained:

- Basic information: Name, blood type, allergies, pre-existing conditions.
- Emergency essentials: Medications, medical device needs, contact lenses.

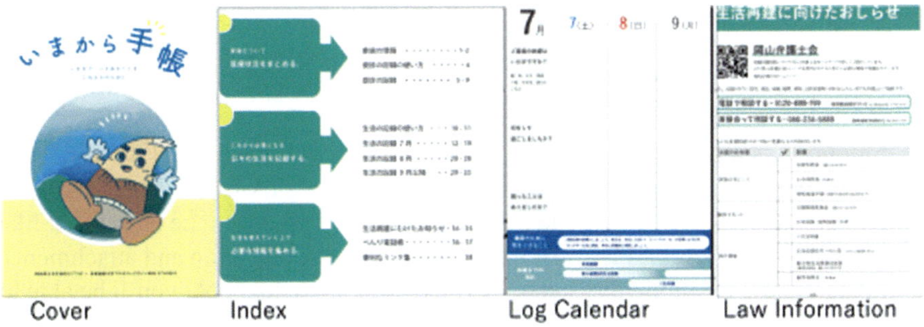

Fig. 7.3 Imakara techo Logbook

- Medical record pages: For documenting consultations during disaster response.
- Seasonal health guidance: "One-word notes" on health risks by time of year.
- Recovery support information: Checklists of available government assistance, QR codes for related websites (in cooperation with local bar associations).
- Diary format pages: For daily health and life event recording.

The logbooks were distributed through multiple channels:

1. First month post-flood: Volunteers distributed "Imakara Logbooks" at evacuation centers and event sites, explaining their use.
2. Four months post-flood: "Korekara Logbooks" distributed during health consultations at promotional events.
3. Ongoing: Available at government offices, announced through mass media.

Between June 2020 and January 2021, a qualitative study was conducted with seven women users (average age 70, range 65–75) who had been affected by the July 2018 floods (Miyamoto et al., 2023). Semi-structured interviews revealed how the logbooks functioned across three dimensions of disaster response.

7.4.2 Functions and Impact

Self-Care

The logbooks served multiple self-care functions:

- Rebuilding record-keeping habits: "I lost the habit of writing recently, but the logbook got me back into writing" (Participant TG-8-1).
- Memory and memoranda: "I recorded what I remembered with the logbook (as a memorandum)" (TC-2-1); "In the logbook, I recorded what I did that day at the office, whom I met, what kind of people I met, my contact information (phone and address), and other details" (TG-9-2).
- Reflective processing: "Despite my age, I have a wealth of experience and wisdom that allow me to make the right choices in my own way" (TF-4-4); "When I was mentally down, I thought it was important to look back and see how things had progressed before reassessing myself" (TF-9-1).
- Action planning: "Writing in a logbook enabled me to plan clearly, rather than vaguely" (TG-7-2); "I would have been going back and forth, unsure what to do if I hadn't written in the logbook" (TG-7-2).
- Emotional support: "The logbook supported me emotionally" (TB-5-1); "The words outside the logbook column made me smile" (TA-6-1); "I kept thinking that the logbook was telling me to stay strong. So I used it to the end. It felt like a companion" (TA-11-1—a striking example of personification and attachment).
- Preparedness for future disasters: "If you record it in a logbook, you'll be able to see your issues and connect them to the next step" (TF-9-1).

Mutual Aid

The logbooks facilitated communication and care coordination:

- Contact restoration: "My contacts and phone book also washed away, and I had nothing left, so the handy phone book helped me a lot" (TB-4-1); "The contact information for the paperwork in the logbook was helpful" (TG-1-3).
- Remembering support: "I wanted to remember the support I received by writing it down" (TA-15-2); "I felt my friends' support" (TG-7-3).

Public Assistance

The logbooks helped maintain social rhythms and cultural continuity:

- Seasonal reminders: "The comments [under the calendar] made me realize that I should not put off the seasonal event (visiting the cemetery) but rather complete it" (TG-7-3); "The logbook helped me remember seasonal events even amid a hectic life" (TG-10-1).

7.4.3 The Logbook as Decentralized Personal Health Record (PHR)

From a health systems perspective, the logbook functioned as a decentralized, analog form of Personal Health Record, allowing evacuees to retain and share critical health information even when digital systems failed or formal medical access was disrupted. This parallels the digital PHR initiatives discussed in Chap. 2 (Naruse on digital inclusion) and Chap. 5 (Hidaka Mura's integrated health information systems), but demonstrates the continued importance of analog resilience in contexts where: Digital infrastructure is compromised, elderly populations have limited digital literacy, simplicity and immediate usability are paramount, and personal ownership and control of health data are essential.

Nurses and support workers used the logbooks as a communication bridge—both to document observations during home visits and to understand residents' evolving needs across the transition from acute evacuation to long-term recovery. Its flexible structure allowed individuals to "write what matters" in their own words, capturing context-sensitive risks and health behaviors in a format usable for both self-care and primary care.

The Imakara/Korekara Logbook offers a replicable model for community-based PHR collection and emotional resilience building under climate-induced disaster conditions. Key design principles include:

1. *Familiarity*: Leveraging a trusted cultural model (Maternal and Child Health Handbook) reduces adoption barriers.
2. *Multi-functionality*: Combining medical records, daily diary, contact information, and emotional reflection in one tool.
3. *Distributed control*: Individuals own their data and decide when/how to share.

4. *Offline resilience*: Paper format ensures accessibility regardless of technological infrastructure.
5. *Emotional significance*: The logbook becomes more than a record—it is a "companion" that provides comfort and motivation.
6. *Integration with care systems*: Designed to be useful for both individual self-management and professional health assessment.

The study's authors concluded: "Even in times of disaster when external support is challenging to obtain, self-care and connections with the local community cultivated during normal times are essential" (Miyamoto et al., 2023). This finding reinforces the book's central argument that resilience is built in peacetime, not improvised in crisis—and that data tools (whether digital maps or paper logbooks) succeed when they amplify existing social capital rather than replacing it.

7.4.4 Reconceptualizing the Logbook: Disaster PHR as Minimum Viable Implementation

Beyond its surface function as a health diary, the Imakara/Korekara Logbook represents a disaster-optimized Personal Health Record—the minimum viable implementation of longitudinal health data portability in extreme conditions. This framing shifts our understanding from "a nice emotional support tool" to "a critical data infrastructure element" with specific design innovations:

- *Solving "assessment fatigue"*: In disaster contexts, affected residents are often subjected to repetitive assessment by multiple agencies—different government departments, NGOs, and health workers each conducting their own intake interviews. This creates:
  - *Emotional exhaustion*: Retelling traumatic experiences multiple times.
  - *Information loss*: Details forgotten or omitted in repeated tellings.
  - *Service gaps*: Lack of coordination means some needs are addressed redundantly while others are missed.

  The logbook externalizes the assessment burden to the individual's control: residents document their information once (or continuously update it), then share selectively with service providers. This transforms the power dynamic from "residents answering the same questions repeatedly" to "residents presenting their self-documented situation on their terms."
- *Data portability without digital infrastructure*: In post-disaster contexts where medical records are destroyed by flooding or fire, or electronic Health Record (EHR) systems are offline due to power outages:
  - Residents are displaced across multiple temporary housing sites, potentially in different municipalities.
  - Healthcare access is fragmented (visiting different mobile clinics, temporary facilities, or out-of-area hospitals).

The logbook becomes the only continuous, portable health data source that follows the individual. Unlike digital PHR systems that require functioning internet, device access, and digital literacy, the paper logbook just works—it requires no charging, no passwords, no training, no infrastructure dependencies.

- *Analog–digital complementarity*: The logbook's value is not in replacing digital systems but in bridging the gap until digital systems are restored and providing a low-tech backup for populations with limited digital access. In the Mabi case, the logbook functioned in parallel with digital initiatives (Mabi Care Map, OpenStreetMap coordination, LINE/Google Forms surveys), each serving complementary roles:
  - Digital systems: Aggregate community-level data, enable real-time coordination, and visualize spatial patterns.
  - Analog logbooks: Capture individual-level longitudinal data, preserve privacy, and ensure accessibility for elderly and digitally excluded populations.

  This complementarity suggests a hybrid data ecosystem model rather than binary digital-versus-analog choices.

7.5 The Mabi Care Map: Participatory Open Data in Action

Amid this information vacuum—10,000 displaced, collapsed infrastructure, no reliable way to know which services functioned—the Mabi Care Map emerged. Catalyzed by the author and local volunteers, the effort employed participatory mapping using OpenStreetMap (OSM) to crowdsource essential survival data: infrastructure status (blocked vs. passable roads), usable toilet and water locations, evacuation center occupancy, and operating hours of surviving pharmacies and stores.

By leveraging OSM's open architecture, volunteers updated data in near real-time as conditions changed. This interactive spatial visualization empowered residents to make informed decisions, transforming abstract uncertainty into actionable knowledge. The Mabi Care Map exemplifies the Health EDRM principle that community participation is central to effective disaster response—particularly when formal systems have collapsed and trust-based, locally embedded information networks become the primary health infrastructure.

Genesis of the Mabi Care Map

It was in this information vacuum that the "Mabi Care Map" initiative emerged as a community-driven lifeline (Mabi Care, 2018). The effort was catalyzed by a disaster nursing specialist from Mabi (the lead author of the project) who happened to be in her hometown during the flood and immediately began coordinating health relief activities. Together with local volunteers, including nurses and civic tech enthusiasts, the team realized that mapping critical resources could empower residents and fill information gaps.

They first identified the essential data needed for daily life and health care in the disaster's aftermath:

- Infrastructure status: Which roads were open or blocked
- Basic necessities: Locations of usable toilets and running water
- Shelter information: Occupancy and capacity of evacuation centers
- Commercial services: Operating hours of nearby convenience stores and pharmacies
- Relief distribution: Points of distribution for relief supplies
- Hygiene facilities: Availability of facilities like public baths or showers
- Isolated communities: Location of areas cut off by the floods
- Real-time disaster indicators: Water levels, inundation extent, levee breaches

These pieces of information—often known only anecdotally or spread by word of mouth—were all crucial for maintaining health and well-being in the days after the flood.

Participatory Mapping Using OpenStreetMap
To gather and disseminate this information systematically, the Mabi Care team turned to a participatory mapping approach using OpenStreetMap (OSM) as its platform (Fig. 7.1). OSM, a free and open-source global mapping tool, allowed the community to create a shared map of the disaster area that anyone could edit and access. This choice was deliberate: by leveraging OSM's open data infrastructure, the map data could be freely used, updated, and redistributed by residents and responders alike.

In essence, the Mabi Care Map was envisioned as a commons—an open information hub created *by* the community *for* the community—to support both mutual aid among residents and more effective assistance from authorities. The use of OSM meant the map could be modified on the fly to reflect changing conditions, and the data (licensed under Creative Commons) could be integrated into other systems or analyses as needed.

Participatory mapping in action: Over the ensuing days and weeks, small teams of volunteers fanned out across the flood-affected neighborhoods to collect field data for the map. They drove or walked through the debris-laden streets with notebooks and GPS-enabled devices, making note of any observable status updates. Health professionals in the group paid special attention to medical and welfare facilities—if a clinic or pharmacy was water-damaged and closed, that would be marked, as would any makeshift first-aid stations or mobile health clinics that arrived.

The volunteers also spoke with residents they encountered, listening to their needs and discovering resources through local knowledge. All this information was then rapidly digitized, geotagged, and uploaded to the Mabi Care Map website in near real-time (Mabi Care, 2018) (Fig. 7.4). The resulting map became an interactive visualization of the community's critical needs and resources: users could open the map on a smartphone or computer and see icons and notes for things like working toilets, available baths, open stores, functioning hospitals, and safe routes through town.

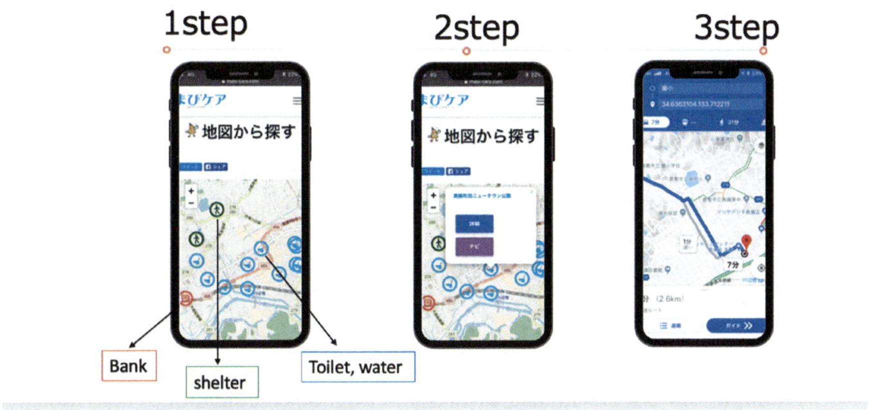

Fig. 7.4 Interface of Mabi Care Map

Box 7.1: Open Data Versus Personal Health Records (PHRs)—Complementary Tools for Community Resilience

A common source of confusion in health informatics and disaster response is the distinction between open data and Personal Health Records (PHRs). While both play crucial roles in empowering communities and supporting health systems, they serve fundamentally different purposes and operate under different governance principles.

Open Data

- Definition: Publicly accessible datasets that can be freely used, modified, and shared by anyone
- Purpose: Enable transparency, collective decision-making, and coordinated action at the population level
- Governance: Published under open licenses (e.g., Creative Commons, Open Data Commons)
- Scope: Aggregated, anonymized, or non-identifiable information about community resources, infrastructure, and public health indicators
- Examples in Mabi: Location of functioning toilets, open pharmacies, evacuation shelter capacity, road accessibility
- Access: Public—anyone can view, download, and use the data
- Privacy concerns: Minimal (data is intentionally de-identified or refers to public infrastructure)

(continued)

Box 7.1 (continued)

Personal Health Records (PHRs)

- Definition: Individual-level health information controlled by the patient/resident
- Purpose: Enable continuity of care, self-management, and informed health decisions for specific individuals
- Governance: Protected by privacy laws (e.g., Japan's Personal Information Protection Act); individual owns and controls access
- Scope: Personal medical history, medications, allergies, chronic conditions, vaccination records, clinical notes
- Examples in Mabi: Imakara/Korekara Logbooks containing individual health status, medication lists, and doctor visit records
- Access: Private—controlled by individual, shared only with trusted care providers or family
- Privacy concerns: High (contains sensitive personal information requiring strong protection)

How They Work Together

The Mabi disaster response demonstrates how these two data types complement each other:

1. Open Data (Mabi Care Map) provided the *environmental context*: "Where can I find medical care? Which routes are safe?"
2. PHR (Imakara Logbook) provided *individual health context*: "What are my chronic conditions? What medications do I need?"
3. Together, they empowered residents to make informed, personalized decisions: An elderly resident with diabetes could use the Care Map to locate an open pharmacy, and use their Logbook to show the pharmacist exactly which insulin they required.

This integration exemplifies patient-centered disaster response: open data creates the infrastructure for informed action, while PHRs ensure that individual health needs are not lost in the chaos. As discussed in Chap. 2 (PHR for digital inclusion) and Chap. 5 (integrated health information systems), both data ecosystems must be designed with equity and trust in mind.

Key Principle: Open data serves the collective; PHR serves the individual. Both require ethical governance, but open data prioritizes transparency while PHR prioritizes privacy.

Box 7.2: The Open Data Workflow for Disaster Response—From Collection to Community Action

One of the critical lessons from the Mabi Care Map is that effective open data initiatives require a systematic workflow that transforms raw observations into actionable community knowledge. This workflow can be adapted for future disasters and integrated into routine community health planning (the "Society 5.0 Nightingale" model).

Phase 1: Data Collection (Field Observation and Crowdsourcing)

Volunteer teams, local nurses, and residents systematically document infrastructure status, health facility operations, resource availability, and vulnerable populations using GPS-enabled devices and paper surveys. The challenge is labor-intensive coordination; best practice involves pre-preparing baseline maps of key facilities during peacetime so volunteers need only update changes during crises.

Phase 2: Data Processing and Standardization

Technical volunteers with GIS skills geocode field notes, standardize data labels (e.g., "clinic-open," "toilet-functional"), and cross-reference crowd-sourced reports with official sources for quality control. Rapid feedback loops, version control, and flagging unverified data help ensure accuracy amid rapidly changing conditions.

Phase 3: Visualization and Dissemination

Web developers and communication specialists create accessible web maps (desktop and mobile), generate printed maps for offline use, and produce summary dashboards for officials and responders. Multi-channel distribution (online + offline) with simple icons and multiple languages addresses the digital divide and ensures equity across populations.

Phase 4: Community Verification and Feedback

Residents and frontline responders test map accuracy in real-world navigation, report errors or outdated information, and identify missing data points or emerging needs. Clearly labeling data timestamps and confidence levels while prioritizing critical corrections maintains trust—essential when errors can be life-threatening.

Phase 5: Decision-Making and Resource Allocation

Local government, healthcare administrators, NGOs, and residents use the map to identify service gaps, prioritize aid distribution, coordinate volunteer deployments, and inform personal evacuation and health decisions. Integrating open data into official response protocols and training government staff in data literacy helps overcome siloed decision-making.

Phase 6: Continuous Update and Learning

Map stewards, academic partners, and community organizations provide real-time updates, conduct post-disaster analysis to identify vulnerability patterns and data gaps, and incorporate lessons into future preparedness plans. Institutionalizing the process—building capacity during peacetime rather than only in emergencies—sustains volunteer energy and secures long-term impact.

(continued)

Box 7.2 (continued)

Connection to "Society 5.0 Nightingales"

This workflow embodies the data stewardship role envisioned for next-generation community nurses: not just care providers, but knowledge brokers who translate lived experience into actionable intelligence; not just technology users, but ethical data governors who balance transparency with privacy; not just disaster responders, but community capacity builders who ensure data skills are distributed, not centralized.

7.6 Challenges and Lessons Learned

The grassroots mapping and community hub initiatives faced interconnected challenges that provide essential lessons for replicating data-driven disaster response models.

Labor intensity and volunteer sustainability emerged as the primary operational challenge. Continuously gathering, verifying, and updating data amid an evolving disaster proved overwhelming, with team members experiencing significant burden. This highlighted the critical need for pre-disaster data preparedness: if baseline maps of health facilities, care homes, and community assets were maintained during peacetime, volunteers could focus on documenting changes ("Clinic X is closed due to flooding") Rather than mapping everything from scratch. Future implementations should integrate disaster planning into routine community health mapping, building capacity before crises occur. The digital divide created immediate access barriers. with power and telecommunications initially down, many residents—particularly elderly populations and those in isolated areas—could not access online maps. The team mitigated this through mobile phone charger distribution and printed map sharing at shelters, demonstrating that multi-channel distribution strategies (online + offline) Must be planned from the outset. Digital-only solutions systematically exclude vulnerable populations precisely when they need support most.

Data accuracy and trust required constant vigilance amid rapidly changing conditions and crowdsourced inputs. The team established rapid feedback loops, cross-checking community reports against official updates when available, and implementing transparency protocols: timestamping all updates, flagging unverified reports, and clearly communicating uncertainty levels. Despite these challenges, the map gained community trust as residents saw their own observations and needs reflected—it became a living repository of local knowledge, not an external imposition. Integration with official systems initially faced institutional unfamiliarity. Local officials were uncertain how to incorporate community-generated open data into formal response protocols. Over time, however, officials began monitoring the publicly available Mabi Care Map, finding it a useful supplement to official information. In some cases, the city later adopted elements of the Mabi Care approach for improving its own disaster data-sharing practices. This gradual institutional learning underscores the necessity of proactive collaboration—joint training exercises, data-sharing agreements, and mutual capacity-building—before disasters occur, not during them. These challenges reveal a fundamental insight: community-driven data initiatives succeed not by replacing official systems, but by creating complementary infrastructure that is trusted, accessible, and responsive to local realities. The next section examines how these lessons translate into measurable empowerment outcomes and sustainable models for community resilience.

7.7 Impact and Analysis: From Data to Health Equity

The Mabi case demonstrates that data-driven community empowerment operates across four interconnected dimensions, each strengthening community capacity to protect health and dignity during crises.

Empowerment Outcome 1: Situational Awareness
The Kanbara Gofukuten shop and Mabi Care Map together created a real-time information commons, where residents, volunteers, and external responders could exchange updates, clarify rumors, and build a shared understanding of evolving conditions. Physical co-location at Kanbara enabled synchronous, multi-directional information flow that digital-only systems could not replicate—especially given power and connectivity constraints. The map extended this awareness spatially, making visible which services functioned, where gaps existed, and who needed urgent support. This transparency transformed chaos into legibility, enabling collective sense-making under extreme uncertainty.

Empowerment Outcome 2: Decision Capacity
Residents gained access to actionable information—which pharmacies had insulin, where functioning toilets existed, which roads were passable—that enabled informed decisions about immediate survival priorities. For example, an elderly resident requiring dialysis could consult the map (or ask a volunteer using it) to identify operational hospitals in neighboring districts. Isolated pockets of people in rural outskirts, previously invisible to formal responders, were pinpointed so outreach teams could deliver supplies and medical care. However, decision capacity was strongest for those who physically accessed the shop or had digital literacy to use online maps; isolated residents or those with mobility constraints remained information-poor unless proactively reached—revealing persistent equity challenges even within community-driven models.

Empowerment Outcome 3: Care Continuity
The Imakara/Korekara Logbook system provided individual-level health tracking that complemented the Mabi Care Map's collective spatial intelligence. Families could

maintain medication records, document symptoms, and communicate health status across fragmented care settings—critical when medical records were destroyed by flooding and usual providers were inaccessible. The shop facilitated informal care coordination (connecting families with volunteer babysitters, linking elderly residents with health workers), though this lacked systematic longitudinal tracking mechanisms. The synergy between analog PHR (logbook) and open data (map) demonstrates that personal and population health data are mutually reinforcing: individual records inform aggregate needs assessment, while spatial visualization guides individual navigation.

Empowerment Outcome 4: Governance Shift

Perhaps most profoundly, these initiatives represented a bottom-up governance transformation. Kanbara Gofukuten—a community member's family shop, not a government agency or formal NGO—became a recognized coordinator and information broker. The Mabi Care Map—created by grassroots volunteers, not official planners—became the authoritative data source for service availability. This challenged hierarchical disaster response norms, demonstrating that legitimacy and effectiveness can emerge from *jimoto* embeddedness rather than formal institutional authority. Local officials initially unfamiliar with community-generated data gradually incorporated it into formal protocols, with some municipalities later adopting Mabi Care elements as templates for their own systems. This institutional learning reveals a pathway: grassroots innovation can catalyze official reform when trust is earned through demonstrated value.

Sustainability and Scalability Challenges

These empowerment outcomes were achieved under extraordinary conditions—a disaster that created both urgent need and temporary social mobilization. Sustaining such initiatives during peacetime requires addressing *three critical dependencies*:

1. *Reliance on "rooted professionals"*: The Kanbara model depended heavily on the author's unique positionality (disaster nursing specialist + local resident + family resources). Scaling this approach requires systematically identifying or developing similar dual-identity actors in other communities—a workforce development challenge explored in Sect. 7.9.
2. *Volunteer burnout and resource constraints*: Data collection, verification, and maintenance are labor-intensive. Without institutionalized support (funding, technical infrastructure, recognition), volunteer energy inevitably wanes post-crisis.
3. *Equity gaps within community-driven systems*: While more responsive than top-down approaches, grassroots initiatives still risk replicating exclusion if marginalized voices (non-Japanese speakers, persons with disabilities, isolated elderly) are not proactively centered in co-design and implementation.

The hotel evacuation pilot (Sect. 7.8) provides a contrasting case: a well-resourced, multi-stakeholder initiative that nonetheless struggled with adoption—revealing that good intentions and technical capacity are insufficient without behavioral insight, cultural alignment, and iterative co-design. Together, the Mabi and Kochi cases illuminate both the potential and the preconditions for data-driven community empowerment.

7.8 The Hotel Evacuation Pilot: Jimoto Sousei Horizontal Deployment as Implementation Science

The success of Mabi's grassroots data initiatives raised a critical question: *Could similar models be proactively designed and deployed in other regions before disasters strike?* The 2021 Kochi hotel evacuation pilot represents an early experiment in *horizontal deployment*—adapting community-driven resilience principles to a new geographic context with different stakeholders, infrastructure, and cultural dynamics. Rather than a "failed intervention," this pilot serves as an essential *implementation science discovery process* that illuminates the gap between technical feasibility and behavioral adoption.

7.8.1 Context and Design: Distributed Evacuation for the COVID-19 Era

By 2021, a pressing challenge had emerged: how to enable safe evacuations when traditional shelters (gymnasiums, community halls) concentrate people in crowded spaces—a grave concern during pandemics. As documented in Sect. 7.3, Mabi's shelters had faced severe overcrowding (2000+ evacuees in facilities designed for 480), creating compound health hazards: heat stress, infectious disease risk, privacy loss, and inadequate accommodation for vulnerable populations. The concept of "*distributed evacuation*"—dispersing people to relatives' homes, cars on high ground, or hotels—offered a promising alternative.

In Kochi Prefecture, a multi-stakeholder consortium developed an *insurance-backed hotel evacuation program*: residents could purchase advance coverage that would subsidize hotel stays if disaster evacuation orders were issued. The pilot involved a nonprofit disaster response organization (coordinator), a major national insurance provider (financial risk coverage), an urban planning research institute (scalability analysis), municipal governments, a local university (disaster nursing specialists, including the author), community disaster preparedness organizations, and two participating hotels in Kochi City.

A pre-pilot survey (October–December 2021) revealed approximately *60% of respondents expressed interest*—a strong signal of perceived need. However, when test sales launched (November–December 2021), uptake was insufficient to proceed with full-scale implementation.

7.8.2 Implementation Barriers: Beyond Stated Preferences

Post-pilot analysis revealed a classic *needs-demand gap*: stated preferences (survey interest) did not translate into revealed preferences (actual purchase behavior). This gap exposed multiple interconnected barriers:

Cognitive barriers: Most residents had never evacuated to a hotel; it existed outside their mental model of disaster response. Without experiential anchors or vivid narratives, hotel evacuation remained abstract and difficult to value.

Complacency paradox: Kochi residents, precisely because they were "used to" typhoons, felt confident in existing coping strategies (staying home on upper floors, evacuating to relatives). Experience bred familiarity, which bred complacency—undermining demand for novel preparedness measures.

Service design challenges: The insurance framing emphasized uncertain future benefit rather than guaranteed peace of mind; complex terms created cognitive load; only two hotels participated, raising capacity and accessibility concerns; transportation logistics (how to reach hotels during active flooding) remained unsolved.

Temporal and communication failures: Launching post-typhoon season (November–December) when disaster salience was low; by late 2021, COVID-19 concerns had ebbed, reducing urgency; many residents simply had not heard about the program.

Target market mismatch: Feedback suggested a stronger appeal as a gift for elderly parents (adult children purchasing coverage) or corporate risk management (companies ensuring employee safety) than as personal purchases—indicating the pilot had marketed to the wrong demographic segment.

7.8.3 Critical Discoveries: What the Pilot Revealed

The hotel evacuation pilot's value lies not in achieving mass adoption, but in *systematically surfacing implementation prerequisites* often invisible in needs assessments:

Discovery 1: Needs ≠ Demand Without Behavioral Design
60% survey interest indicates theoretical recognition of value but reveals nothing about willingness to act. Effective implementation requires behavioral nudges (default options, social proof, experiential learning through trial evacuations), simplified decision-making, and message framing optimization—elements absent from the pilot's design.

Discovery 2: Social Infrastructure Determines Service Uptake
Just as Mabi Care Map succeeded because it was embedded in trusted social networks (Kanbara Gofukuten as information commons), hotel evacuation likely requires *community champions*—respected local figures who model the behavior

and normalize hotel evacuation as a legitimate, mainstream strategy. The pilot's top-down design lacked this grassroots trust infrastructure.

Discovery 3: Integration Trumps Innovation
Rather than a standalone insurance product, hotel evacuation must integrate with existing systems: personal evacuation plans (government-promoted "My Timeline" tool), municipal disaster management (hotels as designated auxiliary shelters with pre-negotiated capacity), employer benefit packages, or senior care service bundles. Isolated innovations struggle; ecosystem integration succeeds.

Discovery 4: Co-Design Is Not Optional
Top-down service design, even when well-intentioned and technically sound, fails to surface latent barriers (mental models, cultural hesitations, logistical obstacles) that only emerge through iterative co-design with end-users. The pilot's limited community engagement meant these barriers were discovered post-launch rather than during development—a costly sequencing error.

7.8.4 Implications for Jimoto Sousei Nursing: Horizontal Deployment Requires Vertical Depth

The contrast between Mabi's success and Kochi's struggles illuminates a paradox: horizontal deployment (scaling across regions) requires vertical depth (deep community embeddedness) in each new context. Jimoto Sousei Nursing cannot be "rolled out" like a standardized product; it must be co-created within each jimoto's unique cultural, social, and institutional landscape.

For Chap. 8*'s governance agenda*, the hotel pilot demonstrates that multi-stakeholder collaboration and technical capacity are insufficient without:

- *Experiential trust-building*: Opportunities for communities to try services, see neighbors succeed, and update mental models through lived experience
- *Behavioral insight integration*: Partnering with behavioral economists, implementation scientists, and cultural anthropologists—not just engineers and insurers
- *Iterative learning structures*: Treating initial pilots as discovery processes, not deployment targets; investing in systematic reflection and adaptation

For nursing practice, the pilot highlights advanced practice nurse (APNs)'potential role as *cultural intermediaries*: professionals who can help communities expand mental models of disaster preparedness while preserving agency and local knowledge. Future iterations should embed APNs as co-designers and cultural translators, not just service providers.

The hotel evacuation case ultimately reinforces a central thesis: *data-driven innovations empower communities only when they emerge from community realities, not when they are imposed upon them.* This learning directly informs Chap. 8's exploration of governance structures, iterative implementation methods, and the educational agenda for cultivating "Society 5.0 Nightingales" capable of navigating this complexity.

7.9 Conclusion: Data, Care, and the Future of Community Resilience

Chapter 7 has argued that integrating planetary health into primary health care through open data is not merely a technical upgrade—it is a cultural and political transformation that requires literacy, ethical safeguards, and institutions willing to share power.

The case of community-led mapping underscores how participatory data practices can improve responsiveness during crises and strengthen long-term recovery and resilience. At the same time, persistent barriers—privacy concerns, data silos, and institutional inertia—remind us that technology alone cannot deliver equity.

The Mabi experience demonstrates that:

- Resilience is built in peacetime, not improvised in crisis.
- Data tools succeed when they amplify existing social capital rather than replacing it.
- Open data and PHR are complementary, not competing—together they empower both collective and individual action.
- Community nurses are essential knowledge brokers, capable of translating between lived experience and systems-level strategy.
- Analog and digital solutions must coexist to ensure equity across generations and contexts.

Chapter 7 has served as a pre-study—demonstrating the potential and limitations of grassroots, data-driven initiatives in disaster contexts. The Mabi Care Map, Kanbara Gofukuten, Imakara Logbook, and hotel evacuation pilot each revealed critical insights about what works, what fails, and why. These initiatives operated largely at the periphery of formal governance—volunteer-driven, temporarily funded, dependent on exceptional individuals (disaster nurses who happened to be local residents), and lacking systematic institutional integration.

Chapter 8 advances from this foundation to examine formalized Community-Based Participatory Research (CBPR) approaches in Kurashiki and Tosa that embed data-driven empowerment within governance structures. Where Chapter 7 showed community-initiated innovations emerging from crisis, Chap. 8 explores how to institutionalize these capabilities through:

- Governance transformation: Formal mechanisms for community voice in health data systems (not just crisis-driven volunteerism).
- Big data integration with health/disaster monitoring: Moving from ad hoc mapping to systematic, longitudinal surveillance systems that link environmental data, health outcomes, and community knowledge.

- Sustainable CBPR infrastructure: Creating lasting partnerships between municipalities, universities, healthcare systems, and residents—rather than episodic crisis responses.

Chapter 8 also addresses the professional development agenda implied by Chap. 7's experiences: if "Society 5.0 Nightingales" are to serve as data stewards, knowledge brokers, and community facilitators, what educational reforms, practice standards, and policy frameworks are needed? The final chapter closes by reframing community-regenerating nursing as a future-oriented discipline of care, evidence, and practical democracy—linking local action in Japan to global agendas for human security and planetary health.

Study Guide Questions

These questions represent the culmination of the competencies developed throughout this book. Chapter 7 presents the Mabi disaster response as a living laboratory where theory meets practice, where global frameworks become local action, and where nurses demonstrate the full scope of Level III advanced practice nursing.

Unlike previous chapters that focused on specific populations or methodologies, Chap. 7 integrates:

- *Open Governance* (Chap. 4)
- *Digital equity and rural empowerment* (Chap. 5)
- *Gender-responsive, participatory methodologies* (Chap. 6)
- *Data-driven decision-making and implementation science*
- The concept of "*Society 5.0 Nightingales*" as nurse-data stewards.

These questions are designed for readers who have absorbed the content of Chaps. 4, 5 and 6 and are now ready to synthesize, innovate, and lead. They do not fit neatly into a single framework because Level III practice transcends frameworks—it requires adaptive expertise, ethical courage, and the capacity to create new models in the face of unprecedented challenges.

Question 1 (Health EDRM Application)

Using the Health Emergency and Disaster Risk Management (Health EDRM) framework applied to Mabi (Sects. 7.3.1, 7.3.2, 7.3.3, 7.3.4, 7.3.5 and 7.3.6), conduct a comprehensive risk analysis of a community you know well, addressing hazard assessment, vulnerability mapping through an intersectional lens, capacity analysis, including the "hazard map paradox," your ethical positionality as insider/outsider, and actionable priorities with measurable outcomes.

Question 2 (Epistemological Framework)

Reflecting on a disaster you have experienced or studied, critically analyze how the "Know Your Enemy, Know Yourself" framework manifests in practice: What systemic blind spots limited understanding of disaster risks? What community assets or informal systems were invisible to outsiders but critical to the response? How does the Mabi Care Map integrate both ways of knowing, and what are the risks of overconfidence in either domain?

Question 3 (Open Data System Design)

Design a community-driven open data initiative for disaster preparedness or response in your context, specifying the information gap you aim to address, technical architecture that ensures accessibility across digital literacy levels, participatory processes for data collection and verification, governance structures for ethical data stewardship, and mechanisms to address the digital divide.

Question 4 (Complementary Data Systems)

Analyze how open data (collective spatial intelligence like Mabi Care Map) and Personal Health Records (individual health tracking like Imakara Logbook) function as complementary rather than competing systems. How do they address different empowerment needs? What infrastructure—social, technical, governance—is required for effective integration?

Question 5 (Community Hub Reconceptualization)

The Kanbara Gofukuten shop served as a "data intake point" and "information commons" during Mabi's disaster response. Critically evaluate this model: Under what conditions can community spaces (shops, libraries, temples) function as trusted hubs for health data and care coordination? What are the dependencies (e.g., "rooted professionals"), sustainability challenges, and equity risks of this grassroots approach?

Question 6 (Implementation Science Insights)

The Kochi hotel evacuation pilot revealed a needs-demand gap: 60% survey interest but minimal actual adoption. Analyze this case through an implementation science lens: What behavioral, cognitive, social, and structural barriers separated stated preferences from revealed preferences? How would you redesign the intervention using co-design principles, behavioral nudges, and integration with existing systems?

Question 7 (Professional Competency Development)

Chapter 7 introduces "Society 5.0 Nightingales" as nurses who are data stewards, knowledge brokers, and community facilitators. Design a competency development plan for yourself or your organization that cultivates: (1) technical skills (GIS, data visualization, health informatics), (2) facilitation and civic engagement abilities, and (3) systems thinking and policy influence capacities. What educational reforms, practice standards, and institutional supports would enable this transformation?

Question 8 (Scalable Framework Design)

Synthesizing lessons from Mabi (success), Kochi hotel evacuation (implementation challenges), and concepts from Chaps. 1, 2, 3, 4, 5, 6 and 7, design a replicable framework for community-driven disaster health governance. Address: core principles (non-negotiable elements), adaptable components (context-specific), multi-stakeholder governance, data ecosystem architecture, sustainability mechanisms, and evaluation approaches that capture both quantitative outcomes and qualitative stories.

Acknowledgments The author expresses profound gratitude to the residents and care recipients of the Mabi District, Kurashiki City, whose resilience in the aftermath of the 2018 Western Japan Floods gave life to every page of this chapter. The author gratefully acknowledges the sustained collaboration and field-based coordination provided by D-Cradle and its community partners in

Kurashiki, with particular appreciation to Takahiro Ando and Masami Oshima for their practical insights and on-the-ground contributions. The author thanks Seiko Imura (research assistant, Kobe City College of Nursing) for her editorial support and reference management. Generative AI tools assisted with structuring and language refinement; all content was critically reviewed and approved by the author.

Author Contributions Conceptualization; methodology; data analysis; theoretical integration; writing—original draft; writing—review and editing: Sakiko Kanbara. Literature search and reference management: research assistant (Seiko Imura). AI-assisted drafting: Generative AI tools were used to support structuring, data narrative, and language refinement under the supervision of Sakiko Kanbara.

References

Das, S. (2019). *Six months since Western Japan flood. Lessons from Mabi.* CWS Japan. https://www.cwsjapan.org/wp-content/uploads/2019/03/Lessons-From-Mabi.pdf.

Japan Meteorological Agency. (2020). *Number of days with less than 1 mm of precipitation per year.* Okayama Prefecture. https://www.pref.okayama.jp/uploaded/life/726941_6627727_misc.pdf; https://www.data.jma.go.jp/obd/stats/data/bosai/report/2018/20180713/20180713.html.

Kanbara, S., Yamagishi, A., & Ozawa, W. (2019). Co-creation and visualization of disaster mitigation care: With the case of torrential rain in western Japan. *Journal of the National Institute of Public Health, 68*(4), 319–328. Retrieved January 22, 2026 from https://www.jstage.jst.go.jp/article/jniph/68/4/68_319/_pdf/-char/ja (in Japanese).

Kurashiki City. (2019). *Report on July 2018 heavy rain disaster response.* https://www.bousai.go.jp/fusuigai/suigai_dosyaworking/pdf/kurashikikensyou.pdf (Japanese).

Mabi Care. (2018). *Disaster reduction information portal.* https://mabi-care.com.

Miyamoto, J., Hatakeyama, N., & Kanbara, S. (2023). Communication for self-care and the role of a logbook on health risk during a flood disaster. *Health Emergency and Disaster Nursing, 10*(1), 29–40. https://doi.org/10.24298/hedn.2022-0001

Nakamura, Y. (2015). International cooperation through maternal and child health (MCH) handbook. *Bulletin of the Japan Society of Pediatrics, 49*, 135–139. (in Japanese).

Sritart, H., Miyazaki, H., Kanbara, S., & Hara, T. (2020). Methodology and application of spatial vulnerability assessment for evacuation shelters in disaster planning. *Sustainability, 12*(18), 7355. https://doi.org/10.3390/su12187355

Beyond Data: Nursing Insight and Technology for Shaping Future Health Care

8

Sakiko Kanbara

8.1 Introduction: Disaster Nursing at the Inflection Point of the Digital Age

Disaster nursing is no longer a specialty confined to rare, exceptional events. Under planetary health disruption, disasters are becoming chronic conditions of society: recurrent heat waves, seasonal floods, climate-induced displacement, cascading infrastructure failures, and NATECH (Natural-Technological) accidents increasingly intersect with aging populations, chronic disease burdens, socioeconomic inequality, and misinformation epidemics. The traditional distinction between "normal" health care and "disaster" response has eroded—what were once exceptional circumstances are now recurring realities requiring sustained preparedness and adaptive capacity.

This chapter argues that the decisive capability for disaster-resilient health systems is not computational power or technological sophistication but governance-ready relational capacity: the ability to co-design decisions with communities, preserve dignity under pressure, and act decisively without sacrificing fairness or transparency. As Shaw (2020) documents in his analysis of 30 years of science, technology, and academia in disaster risk reduction, the field has evolved from advisory roles—where experts inform policymakers from a distance—to co-designing and co-delivering solutions in partnership with affected communities. This transformation reflects a fundamental recognition that technical knowledge alone cannot address the complex social, cultural, and political dimensions of disaster resilience. Planetary health and syndemic risks make a place clinically decisive in ways that transcend traditional epidemiology. Disaster risks are not experienced by communities as abstract statistical indices or probability distributions. They are experienced

S. Kanbara (✉)
Faculty of Nursing, Kobe City College of Nursing, Kobe, Japan
e-mail: s-kanbara@kobe-ccn.ac.jp

S. Kanbara (ed.), *Transformative Community Health Nursing*,
https://doi.org/10.1007/978-3-032-24405-5_8

as disrupted healthcare access when roads flood, deteriorating shelter conditions that amplify infectious disease transmission, medication shortages when supply chains break, and social isolation when communication networks fail. Understanding disaster vulnerability requires understanding the specific geography, infrastructure, social networks, and cultural practices of each community—what we term the "first mile" of disaster risk reduction.

Complex, cascading disasters—including NATECH-type events where natural hazards trigger technological failures, as demonstrated catastrophically in the 2011 Fukushima nuclear accident—require integrated risk thinking across health, infrastructure, and social systems rather than siloed response plans. The earthquake triggered the tsunami, which caused the power failure, which led to the cooling system breakdown, which resulted in the nuclear meltdown—a cascade that no single-hazard response plan could adequately address. Disaster nursing in this context must cultivate systems thinking: recognizing that health outcomes emerge from complex interactions among individuals, communities, built environments, ecosystems, and governance structures. The digital era amplifies both capacity and harm in disaster contexts. Better situational awareness is technologically possible through real-time data streams, social media monitoring, and geographic information systems. However, surveillance, exclusion, and algorithmic bias can widen vulnerability if digital systems are deployed without governance guardrails. Communities that lack digital access become invisible in data-driven response systems. Algorithmic triage tools trained on the majority populations may systematically disadvantage minorities. Surveillance technologies deployed during emergencies may persist afterward, normalizing intrusive monitoring. Therefore, the fundamental question shifts from "How do we use data to improve disaster response?" to "For whom do we use data, under what governance structures, with what transparency obligations, and accountable to which communities?"

Transformative community health nursing must develop the operational capacity to span the entire disaster management continuum: pre-disaster preparedness that builds community capacity before crises strike, acute response that maintains care quality under chaos, protracted recovery arcs that may extend for years or decades, and long-term transformation that addresses root vulnerabilities rather than merely reconstructing pre-disaster systems. This continuum thinking distinguishes disaster nursing from emergency medicine's focus on acute stabilization—disaster nursing encompasses prevention, structural vulnerability reduction, community empowerment, and systemic transformation. To clarify what this book has already constructed as the foundation for this transformation, we first synthesize Chapters 1, 2, 3, 4, 5, 6 and 7 as an integrated disaster resilience architecture before advancing to the specific methodologies and policy implications of disaster nursing in the digital age.

8.2 Synthesis: What Chaps. 1–7 Have Built for Disaster Resilience

This volume has progressively assembled the core components of disaster resilience from a nursing perspective, positioning human security as the ethical baseline, open governance as the decision architecture, and inclusion as a safety requirement rather than merely an aspirational moral principle. Chapter 8 consolidates these foundational components into a coherent, implementable disaster nursing methodology for the digital age—usable by APNs, educators, researchers, and policymakers across Asia and applicable with appropriate adaptation to diverse global contexts.

Human security, as developed in Chap. 1, reframes disasters not merely as threats to biological survival but as comprehensive assaults on human dignity and agency. This perspective expands nursing's traditional unit of care from individual patients to entire health systems and the social determinants that shape population health. When disasters strike, the immediate threat may be physical injury or disease, but the deeper harms often include loss of livelihood, destruction of social networks, erosion of cultural continuity, and psychological trauma from helplessness. Disaster nursing grounded in human security recognizes that effective response requires addressing these multiple dimensions simultaneously, understanding that sustainable recovery depends on restoring not just physical health but agency, dignity, and community capacity for collective action.

Open governance, elaborated in Chaps. 2 and 3, operationalizes legitimacy by making decisions about resource allocation, shelter management, and data practices transparent, contestable, and participatory. In disasters, trust is not an abstract value but an operational infrastructure. When communities trust that early warnings are accurate and intended to protect them rather than control them, evacuation compliance improves. When shelter residents trust that resource distribution is fair and decisions are made transparently, cooperation increases and conflict decreases. When data collection is governed by clear consent protocols and communities retain ownership of information about their vulnerabilities, participation in risk assessment improves. Open governance transforms trust from an intangible social capital into measurable, cultivable infrastructure that directly impacts disaster outcomes.

The Four Opens framework from Chap. 2 takes on particular urgency in disaster contexts. *Open Mind* requires disaster nursing to acknowledge the limits of professional expertise and remain genuinely open to community knowledge, including traditional risk-reduction practices that may lack scientific validation but encode generations of practical wisdom. *Open Professionalism* demands that nurses operate as facilitators and brokers rather than top-down experts, recognizing that communities possess irreplaceable knowledge about their own vulnerabilities, capacities, and priorities. *Open Data* means making risk information, resource inventories, and decision rationales accessible to communities in formats they can actually use—not just technical reports archived on government websites. *Open Governance* institutionalizes these commitments through formal mechanisms: participatory disaster planning committees, transparent resource allocation protocols, and grievance procedures when communities believe decisions are unjust or exclusionary.

Diversity management and transcultural competence, examined in Chaps. 3 and 4, are not peripheral "soft skills" in disaster contexts—they are operational safety measures critical for risk communication and service continuity. Multilingual early warning systems can mean the difference between timely evacuation and preventable death for non-dominant language speakers. Cultural competence in shelter design—understanding privacy norms, food preferences, religious practices, and gender-specific needs—directly impacts whether vulnerable populations will use shelters or instead remain in dangerous locations. Transcultural nursing recognizes that disaster preparedness and response must be designed from the outset for the actual diversity of the population, not retrofitted afterward when exclusions become undeniable.

Gender equity and social cohesion, analyzed in Chap. 6, are structural determinants of who can evacuate, who can access timely information, and who becomes systematically invisible in disaster statistics, shelter management, and recovery policies. Gender-disaggregated data consistently show that women, especially those with caregiving responsibilities for children or elderly family members, face distinct evacuation barriers. Pregnant and postpartum women require specialized medical support that generic shelter plans often omit. Gender-based violence increases in crowded, poorly designed shelters lacking privacy and security. Yet women are often excluded from disaster planning committees where these issues could be addressed proactively. Gender-responsive disaster nursing means not just acknowledging these patterns but actively redesigning systems to address them: gender-balanced planning committees, shelter designs that protect privacy and safety, care support for family caregivers, and post-disaster services that recognize and address gender-based violence.

Citizen science demonstrated through the Mabi Care Map case in Chap. 7, enables "first mile" intelligence generation where residents become active co-producers of situational awareness rather than passive recipients of expert assessments. Community-based data collection—mapping vulnerable populations, documenting local infrastructure weaknesses, identifying informal mutual aid networks—provides granular, context-specific information that official surveys typically miss. When residents participate in creating risk maps, they develop ownership of the data and a deeper understanding of their community's vulnerabilities. When disaster strikes, these same residents are better prepared to act on the information they helped generate. Citizen science transforms disaster preparedness from a top-down technocratic exercise into a participatory capacity-building process.

These five conceptual pillars—human security, open governance, diversity competence, gender equity, and citizen science—converge to create a disaster nursing paradigm fundamentally different from conventional emergency response models. Rather than expert-driven, protocol-based, top-down intervention, this paradigm positions nurses as facilitators of community resilience, brokers between professional knowledge and local wisdom, and stewards of data governance systems that protect rather than exploit vulnerable populations. With this integrated foundation established, we can now examine how spatial computing transforms disaster data from abstract information into shared situational awareness that enables faster, more legitimate consensus under pressure.

8.3 Spatial Computing for Disaster Nursing: From Explanation to Shared Situation Awareness

In disaster contexts, information often fails not because it is unavailable but because it is not actionable in the lived spaces where decisions must be made. Emergency managers may possess detailed hazard maps and resource inventories, but if affected communities cannot access, interpret, or trust this information, it remains operationally useless. Spatial computing addresses this translation gap by shifting nursing informatics from screen-based dashboards viewed by professionals in distant command centers to space-based decision support embedded in the actual environments where risks manifest and resources must be deployed. For disaster nursing, spatial computing is not merely "cool technology" or a visualization enhancement—it is consensus infrastructure. By representing risks, resources, and constraints in geographic space that stakeholders can see, touch, and navigate together, spatial computing enables multi-perspective simulation and dramatically improves both the quality and speed of collective decision-making under uncertainty. When diverse stakeholders—residents, healthcare workers, emergency managers, community organization leaders—view the same spatial representation of a disaster scenario, they develop shared situational awareness that transcends linguistic and technical barriers. And this is extremely critical, because by reviewing local maps together and discussing disaster preparedness from the prevention stage, we can mitigate damage when disasters strike. Appendix A provides a checklist useful for these discussions.

Participatory mapping serves dual purposes in disaster preparedness and response. Before disasters, participatory mapping exercises identify who is at risk in specific locations, where access breaks occur (impassable roads, bridges with weight limits, and stairs blocking wheelchair users), and which routes and hubs are most likely to fail first under different hazard scenarios.

During disasters, these same spatial databases enable rapid resource deployment by showing exactly where vulnerable populations are located, which evacuation routes remain passable, and where medical supplies and healthcare personnel are most urgently needed. Community participation in map creation ensures accuracy and builds local capacity—residents know their neighborhoods better than any external expert and can identify vulnerabilities that official data miss. Scenario simulation using augmented reality, virtual reality, or even low-tech role-play exercises allows diverse stakeholders to experientially understand constraints they might otherwise overlook. Emergency planners without disabilities often design evacuation routes without considering wheelchair navigation or visual impairments. Healthcare administrators who are not fluent in the dominant language may not grasp how terrifying disasters become when critical information is linguistically inaccessible. Shelter designers without childcare experience may not recognize the impossibility of evacuating with infants without cribs, diapers, and formula. Experiential scenario simulation—whether through VR goggles, wheelchairs pushed through proposed evacuation routes, or role-playing limited language comprehension—generates empathy and understanding that abstract briefings cannot achieve. Before crises force improvisation, scenario simulation reveals design flaws that can be corrected at low cost.

Impact-based early warning represents a fundamental evolution in disaster communication. Traditional early warnings communicated hazard parameters—earthquake magnitude, typhoon wind speeds, and rainfall accumulation. While scientifically precise, these metrics remain abstract to most people who lack the expertise to translate them into personal risk and appropriate protective action. Impact-based early warning translates hazard parameters into place-specific consequences that communities can understand and act upon, like this: "This rainfall will cause the Yoshii River to overflow, flooding the municipal hospital's first floor and cutting off access to the dialysis center. If you require dialysis, evacuate to the designated alternate facility now." By making the consequences concrete and spatially specific, impact-based warning improves both understanding and response. However, spatial computing tools must be designed with robust governance guardrails to prevent transforming care infrastructure into surveillance infrastructure. The same GIS databases that enable rapid resource deployment during disasters could enable permanent monitoring of vulnerable populations if governance protections fail. Location-tracking capabilities that help emergency responders find isolated elderly residents during disasters could normalize intrusive surveillance if extended to non-emergency periods. Consent protocols must clearly specify what data are collected, who can access them, for what purposes, and what happens to the data after emergencies end. Communities must retain meaningful control and oversight—not merely be informed but genuinely empowered to contest inappropriate uses.

For APNs, spatial reasoning must evolve from a specialized skill to a core clinical competency. Understanding how symptoms, exposures, and service disruptions map onto the same geography becomes essential for population health management under crisis conditions. An APN managing shelter healthcare needs spatial awareness of where specific populations are located (dialysis patients, insulin-dependent diabetics, and asthma patients in high-pollution zones), where healthcare resources are available, and what routes connect needs to resources. This spatial clinical competency enables APNs to function as system designers who can rapidly reorganize care delivery when normal infrastructure fails, rather than remaining dependent on institutional structures that may collapse under disaster stress. Yet spatial intelligence alone remains insufficient for legitimate disaster decisions. Even perfect situational awareness cannot determine whether to prioritize scarce resources for the most critically ill or distribute them equitably across all affected populations. Technical knowledge cannot resolve whether to mandate evacuations, overriding individual autonomy, or respect personal choice even when medically dangerous. Risk decisions require not just information but a values compass—which is precisely where culture-led development becomes essential in disaster nursing methodology.

8.4 Culture-Led Development: Values as the Compass of Disaster Preparedness and Recovery

Disaster resilience efforts fail repeatedly—despite technical sophistication and substantial resource investment—when plans ignore what communities actually value and how people actually live. Culture-led development means starting from "what counts as good" in specific community contexts and designing technologies, shelter arrangements, evacuation procedures, and healthcare services accordingly. This is not "localization" as an afterthought or superficial adaptation of predetermined interventions. It is a fundamental methodological commitment: values must guide design from the inception, not be accommodated afterward when plans prove culturally incompatible and compliance fails.

In Asia's profoundly diverse contexts—spanning thousands of languages, dozens of major religious traditions, vastly different kinship systems and household structures, and cultural practices ranging from collective decision-making to hierarchical authority—this values-first approach is not merely good practice but a requirement for equitable survival, governance legitimacy, and sustained recovery. Disaster plans designed for nuclear families fail for extended multi-generational households. Evacuation shelter designs based on individual privacy norms may be inappropriate for cultures where privacy is defined at the family or household levels. Healthcare consent procedures assuming individual autonomy may conflict with cultures where family elders or community leaders appropriately participate in medical decisions.

Local and traditional knowledge must be validated and acknowledged as legitimate expertise, neither romanticized as pristine wisdom nor dismissed as unscientific folklore. Traditional knowledge about disaster risks often encodes practical wisdom accumulated over generations of lived experience. Earthquake-resistant construction techniques developed through centuries of trial and error in seismically active regions may lack engineering documentation but perform remarkably well. Traditional typhoon forecasting based on natural indicators—specific cloud formations, animal behaviors, changes in wind patterns—may provide earlier community-level warnings than official systems. Medicinal plants used for centuries to treat common disaster-related ailments (contaminated water diarrhea, stress-related insomnia, and wound infections) may offer practical low-cost alternatives when pharmaceutical supply chains break. Validating traditional knowledge requires rigorous documentation, scientific testing when feasible, and explicit acknowledgment in disaster plans rather than passive tolerance. When official disaster plans incorporate traditional indicators alongside scientific monitoring, communities experience their knowledge as valued rather than merely tolerated. When shelter designs incorporate traditional healing practices (space for prayer, traditional medicine preparation), residents feel culturally safe rather than alienated. This cultural validation is not sentimentality—it directly impacts compliance, trust, and psychological resilience during prolonged displacements.

Cultural norms fundamentally shape evacuation decisions through mechanisms that disaster planners often overlook. Privacy norms influence whether families will evacuate to communal shelters. Shame about accepting help affects whether vulnerable individuals will self-identify their needs. Family obligation—particularly expectations that adult children care for elderly parents—determines who can evacuate independently and who remains in dangerous locations to fulfill caregiving duties. Gender norms about appropriate behavior in public spaces influence women's willingness to evacuate to mixed-gender shelters. These cultural factors are not irrational barriers to overcome through education but legitimate values that disaster systems must accommodate through design. Shelter design provides concrete examples of culture-led development in practice. Gender-segregated spaces, religiously appropriate food preparation areas, private family sleeping quarters, and facilities for traditional hygiene practices are not luxury amenities but baseline requirements for culturally safe shelter. When shelters fail to provide these features, vulnerable populations—especially women, religious minorities, and families with young children—often refuse to evacuate, remaining in physically dangerous locations they perceive as culturally safer than culturally alien shelters. Recovery transcends physical reconstruction to encompass restoration of agency, social ties, and cultural continuity—core determinants of mental health and long-term resilience that infrastructure-focused recovery plans often neglect. Communities derive identity and meaning from specific places, social rituals, and cultural practices. When disasters destroy not just buildings but community gathering spaces, religious sites, and landscapes imbued with cultural meaning, the psychological harm extends far beyond physical losses. Recovery planning must intentionally support cultural continuity: rebuilding spaces for traditional practices, maintaining social festivals and gatherings even in temporary shelters, preserving cultural heritage even when economically "inefficient," and ensuring that long-term housing solutions accommodate cultural needs for extended family proximity and community connection. Appendix B is a helpful tool to design culture-led disaster preparation/recovery plans.

Technology adoption is ultimately a cultural decision, not a technical problem with social barriers. If digital tools undermine dignity by treating people as data points rather than human beings, if surveillance technologies erode the autonomy that communities value, or if communication platforms exclude those without smartphones or Internet access, these technologies will fail precisely when they are most needed—during the chaos of disaster response when trust and cooperation are essential. Culture-led design prevents techno-solutionism by forcing explicit ethical questions before deployment: Does this technology strengthen or erode community dignity? Does this data system build solidarity or enable stigmatization? Whose values are embedded in this "objective" algorithm? To translate these cultural and narrative realities into disaster response actions without erasing the meaning and context that make them intelligible, disaster nursing requires a distinct methodological capability: the craft of empathy translation that preserves human stories while enabling collective action under resource constraints and time pressure.

8.5 Social Artistry: Empathy-to-Data Translation in Disaster Nursing

Disaster nursing repeatedly confronts a profound dilemma: the most critical information for effective response is often qualitative, contextual, and emotionally charged—yet operational decisions require prioritization, resource allocation, and documentation in forms that health systems and emergency management can process. For example, an elderly resident tearfully explains why she cannot evacuate: fear of abandoning her pet, shame about burdening neighbors, memories of previous shelter trauma, pride in her independence despite obvious frailty. This narrative contains vital clinical information (psychological state, social support deficits, and trauma history) and operational insights (barriers to evacuation compliance), yet transforming it into actionable intelligence risks stripping away the dignity, context, and nuance that make the story intelligible and the person visible. Appendix C below is an Interview Guide, with several key communication examples.

Social artistry is the disciplined craft of translating empathy into data without eroding human dignity. It is not persuasion aimed at changing people's minds or convincing them to comply with expert recommendations. It is a legitimate practice grounded in a fundamental principle: people must be able to recognize themselves in the data that govern them. When quantitative risk scores and resource allocation decisions feel alien and disconnected from people's lived reality, trust collapses and systems fail regardless of their technical sophistication. When communities see their stories and values reflected in how decisions are made and explained, legitimacy increases even when specific outcomes disappoint.

Narratives reveal hidden constraints that quantitative surveys systematically miss. "I'm fine," stated by an elderly resident refusing evacuation may encode multiple intersecting factors: fear of shelter stigma ("only weak people need help"), profound distrust of government authorities based on historical experiences, unspoken disabilities she's concealing to avoid being institutionalized, or cultural obligations to remain and protect the family home. Each of these factors changes the clinical risk assessment and appropriate intervention. Social artistry means developing the interviewing skills, cultural competence, and time investment to hear what remains unspoken, recognizing that silence often carries more meaning than explicit statements.

Translation methodology must preserve silence, ambiguity, and uncertainty as legitimate data signals rather than treating them as noise to be eliminated through better survey design. Mental health assessment, protection from gender-based violence, and identification of exploitation risks all depend on recognizing that what people do not say often matters more than what they do say. A woman who hesitates when asked if she feels safe, changes the subject when asked about her living situation, or gives inconsistent answers about injury causes is providing vital information through her silences and contradictions. Recording these ambiguities explicitly—rather than forcing false clarity—enables better clinical judgment and more appropriate protective interventions. Visual co-design methodologies—collaborative mapping, storyboarding, and dashboard prototyping—provide structured processes through which communities can validate whether quantitative outputs still reflect lived reality. When disaster planners create resource allocation models based on vulnerability indices, presenting the results through interactive maps enables residents to identify errors ("this area isn't actually high risk because we have strong mutual aid networks"), correct missing data ("you've missed all the homebound elderly on this street"), and challenge value judgments ("why are you prioritizing faster hospital access over maintaining community ties?"). This validation process is not merely quality control—it is co-design that generates ownership and legitimacy.

Feedback loops must return analyses and decisions to residents for reinterpretation before finalizing implementation. The technical term "feedback loop" undersells its importance—this is actually a governance mechanism ensuring that expert analysis remains accountable to lived experience. When data analysis reveals unexpected patterns (certain neighborhoods show low evacuation compliance despite high hazard exposure), returning the finding to community representatives often generates explanations that radically reframe interpretation (evacuation routes pass through gang territories, making them dangerous for specific populations). Without this feedback, experts would misdiagnose the problem (lack of awareness) and prescribe ineffective solutions (more education) while missing the actual barrier (unsafe routes). This prevents what we term "data divorce"—the decoupling of quantitative analysis from qualitative reality that produces technically sophisticated but operationally useless outputs. Data divorce occurs when analysts optimize models against metrics that communities do not recognize as important, when resource allocation follows efficiency criteria that communities consider unfair, or when expert risk assessments contradict local knowledge without explaining why the discrepancy exists. Preventing data divorce requires sustained engagement: presenting drafts, soliciting criticism, incorporating feedback, and making explicit when expert judgment must override community preferences (and explaining why).

In crisis operations, social artistry directly supports triage ethics and risk communication. When medical resources are insufficient for all who need them, allocation decisions must be not only medically sound but explainable and defensible to communities experiencing the tragedy of scarcity. Purely utilitarian triage (save the most lives) may violate cultural values about respecting elders or prioritizing children. Purely egalitarian approaches (lottery systems) may feel cruelly random. Social artistry means working with community representatives to establish triage principles before crises, incorporating cultural values about fairness, and ensuring that the rationale for specific decisions can be communicated in ways that maintain trust even under unbearable circumstances. This methodological sophistication in empathy translation becomes operational only when anchored in a concrete unit of practice—the community as the first mile of resilience, where abstract principles become embodied actions and where vulnerability and capacity are negotiated through daily interactions, not crisis interventions.

8.6 Jimoto as the First Mile of Community Resilience

In this chapter, Jimoto is positioned not as a rebranding of community health nursing nor as an exclusively Japanese model requiring adoption elsewhere, but as a Japanese articulation of a universal disaster resilience principle: the first mile of risk reduction is the community's lived environment, where vulnerabilities, capacities, and obligations are negotiated daily through mundane interactions that become critical during crises. Place matters profoundly because disasters do not begin with hazard impact—they begin with pre-existing inequities, fragile infrastructure, weak social cohesion, and institutional failures that leave populations exposed and unprepared.

Shaw's (2020) analysis emphasizes the paradigm shift from "last mile" service delivery—where communities are endpoints passively receiving expert solutions—to "first mile" thinking, where communities define problems, identify priorities, and co-design solutions from the outset with professional facilitation rather than professional dominance. This inversion fundamentally restructures the relationship between nursing expertise and community knowledge. In last-mile approaches, nurses arrive with predetermined protocols and "best practices" derived from other contexts, implementing them with varying degrees of community consultation. In first-mile approaches, nurses arrive with methodological expertise and facilitation capabilities, helping communities articulate their own risks, leverage their own knowledge, and build their own solutions with external support where needed.

The Science Council of Japan's Jimoto Sousei Nursing proposal defines Jimoto as "the home community—geographic or characteristic-based—where residents share exposure to risks and hold collective responsibility for each other's wellbeing" (SCJ, 2020). This definition intentionally avoids rigid geographic boundaries, recognizing that meaningful communities can be spatial (a neighborhood, a municipality, and an island) or relational (migrants sharing language and cultural practices, persons with specific health conditions connecting through support networks, and displaced populations maintaining identity through diaspora connections). What matters is shared exposure and shared decision rights: people affected by the same risks participating meaningfully in decisions about how those risks are managed.

Jimoto-oriented practice matters because it acknowledges that disasters are fundamentally local experiences. National disaster statistics aggregating impacts across entire countries erase the radical heterogeneity of disaster exposure and resilience capacity. A typhoon making landfall may devastate coastal fishing villages while leaving inland cities relatively unscathed. Urban neighborhoods 5 km apart may experience radically different impacts based on building quality, drainage infrastructure, and social cohesion. Rural communities with aging populations face fundamentally different evacuation challenges than urban centers with young demographics. Effective disaster nursing must operate at the scale where these differences are visible and actionable—the scale of the Jimoto.

Community resilience grows through everyday governance practices long before disasters strike: who participates in community meetings, whose voices are heard and valued, who can access municipal services and health information, and whose needs remain invisible in official planning. Strong governance practices—transparent decision-making, inclusive participation, accountable institutions—build social capital that becomes operational capacity during disasters. Communities where residents regularly interact across differences, where local government responds to complaints, and where mutual aid networks function routinely can mobilize these capacities rapidly when crises occur. Communities where governance is opaque, participation is limited to elites, and trust is low struggle to coordinate an effective response even when physical infrastructure remains intact.

University-community partnerships for disaster resilience must be institutionalized rather than remaining dependent on ad hoc projects or individual faculty enthusiasm. Disaster resilience requires continuity measured in years and decades, not the 2–3 year cycles of typical research grants. Building trust between universities and communities takes time. Participatory research developing local knowledge requires sustained engagement. Training community health workers and building local organizational capacity cannot be accomplished through brief interventions. Institutionalizing these partnerships—through formal memoranda of understanding, dedicated university positions, ongoing funding streams, and integration into academic curricula—ensures continuity when individual faculty retire or move.

Place-based knowledge becomes globally transferable through rigorous documentation that separates context-specific details from generalizable principles. The Kochi Prefecture disaster mitigation care model succeeds in its specific context through particular interventions (pre-positioned medication supplies, pet-friendly shelters, and GIS mapping of vulnerable populations). Other communities facing similar challenges (aging populations, earthquake/tsunami risks, and rural geography) can learn from Kochi—not by copying specific interventions but by adapting the underlying methodology: participatory vulnerability assessment, community co-design of solutions, spatial visualization of risks and resources, governance protocols balancing privacy and life-saving information sharing. This is an exporting method, not exporting "Japanese solutions"—recognizing that Jimoto Sousei Nursing's value lies in its methodological rigor and community-centered epistemology, not in specific techniques that may transfer poorly to different contexts.

Thus, Jimoto functions best as the platform where disaster nursing becomes preventive (addressing vulnerabilities before hazards strike), participatory (engaging communities as co-designers), and transformative (building capacity rather than creating dependency). The Kochi model demonstrates these principles through a six-step cycle: vulnerability mapping identifying specific at-risk populations, participatory assessment surfacing unstated needs, collaborative solution design addressing cultural barriers to evacuation, spatial visualization making abstract risks concrete, governance protocols establishing trust through transparency, and continuous improvement through drills and post-event evaluations.

Having established Jimoto as the first-mile unit of practice, we must now articulate how disaster nursing's responsibilities align with international frameworks that have evolved over three decades of disaster risk-reduction scholarship and practice, particularly the science-to-action agenda that has emerged from the Sendai Framework and regional implementation efforts.

8.7 From "Science of What" to "Science of How": A Sendai/Bangkok-Aligned Science-to-Action Agenda for Disaster Nursing

Sendai Framework (2015–2030) has progressively shifted emphasis toward solution-driven, implementation-based science—what Shaw terms the "science of how." This paradigm shift reflects hard-won recognition that producing knowledge is necessary but insufficient for disaster risk reduction. Communities overwhelmed by hazards do not primarily need more research documenting their vulnerability—they need implementable solutions co-designed to fit their specific contexts, resources, and values. Researchers and practitioners must move beyond advisory roles where experts inform policymakers from a distance, toward co-designing and co-delivering solutions in sustained partnership with affected communities. This transformation has profound implications for disaster nursing, clarifying what a flagship disaster nursing agenda must carry beyond clinical emergency response: governance-ready knowledge production aligned with international frameworks, evidence dissemination in forms communities and policymakers can actually use, continuous monitoring and learning from both drills and real events, and systematic capacity building through first-mile co-design and co-delivery.

The Sendai Framework for Disaster Risk Reduction 2015–2030 (UN, 2015) provides the authoritative global policy architecture for disaster risk reduction, emphasizing four priorities for action: understanding disaster risk, strengthening disaster risk governance, investing in disaster risk reduction for resilience, and enhancing disaster preparedness for effective response and better recovery. The Bangkok Principles for the implementation of the health aspects of the Sendai Framework (UNDRR & WHO, 2016) specifically elaborate how health systems, including nursing, should operationalize these priorities. Together, these frameworks provide a science-to-action roadmap for disaster nursing that replaces generic role descriptions with concrete, internationally aligned responsibilities.

8.7.1 Assess and Update: Dynamic Risk Intelligence

Disaster nursing must systematically incorporate disaster-related mortality, morbidity, and disability data into multi-hazard early warning systems, health core indicators, and national/subnational risk assessments (Bangkok Principle 1). This is not passive data collection but active intelligence generation, recognizing that risk landscapes change continuously. New urban developments alter flood patterns. Aging demographics shift health system demand during disasters. Climate change makes historical hazard patterns obsolete. Migration changes community demographics and linguistic requirements. Keeping risk maps and vulnerability assessments current for these dynamic, cascading hazards requires sustained institutional commitment, not episodic studies. This continuous assessment responsibility demands that disaster nursing develop sustained surveillance capacity integrating multiple data sources: routine healthcare utilization patterns revealing baseline vulnerability, environmental monitoring detecting hazard evolution, infrastructure assessments identifying system fragilities, and social network analysis mapping mutual aid capacity. APNs functioning as local intelligence nodes can synthesize these diverse signals, recognizing patterns that centralized systems miss—the clustering of medication-dependent patients in specific neighborhoods, the erosion of social cohesion following economic disruptions, the emergence of misinformation undermining trust in official warnings.

8.7.2 Disseminate: Evidence Translation for Action

Producing sophisticated risk analyses that remain trapped in academic journals or technical reports fails the science-to-action mandate. Disaster nursing must build accessible risk databases in partnership with professional bodies and academic societies, translating evidence into actionable guidance for policymakers, practitioners, and residents (Bangkok Principle 2). This translation work requires multiple formats and communication channels: technical briefings for policymakers requiring evidence to justify resource allocation, practical protocols for frontline health workers needing decision support under pressure, and community-accessible materials in multiple languages and literacy levels explaining what risks exist and what protective actions are feasible. The Japan Society of Disaster Nursing's systematic synthesis of research findings into practical guidance documents (Miyamae, 2023) exemplifies this dissemination responsibility. Rather than expecting policymakers or practitioners to read hundreds of individual studies, professional societies curate evidence, identify consensus findings and remaining controversies, and produce synthesis documents that busy decision-makers can actually use. Disaster nursing research that fails to support this synthesis and dissemination function—remaining instead in technical silos accessible only to specialists—abdicates the science-to-action commitment.

8.7.3 Monitor and Review: Learning Systems

Continuous evaluation of whether health is systematically integrated into disaster risk reduction (DRR) frameworks, plans, and policies—using inequity-sensitive nursing indicators and revising plans after both drills and real events—operationalizes organizational learning (Bangkok Principle 3). This is not compliance monitoring, checking whether plans exist on paper, but a substantive assessment of whether plans actually work when tested. Mock evacuation drills reveal whether wheelchair-accessible routes exist in reality or only in plans. Tabletop exercises are surfacing conflicts between emergency protocols and normal healthcare regulations. Post-event reviews documenting what worked, what failed, and why—not to assign blame but to improve future response. Monitoring requires establishing measurable indicators that capture not just disaster outcomes (deaths, injuries, and economic losses) but also equity and governance quality. Were vulnerable populations reached by early warnings? Did resource distribution reflect actual need or institutional convenience? Were decisions made transparently with meaningful community participation? These governance indicators provide early warning of systemic failures before they manifest in disaster casualties. Communities excluded from planning will be excluded from response, but this becomes measurable only if monitoring explicitly tracks participation and inclusion.

8.7.4 Capacity Building: Systematic Professional Development

Integrating DRR into health education and field training, cultivating disaster nursing specialists with interdisciplinary competence, and enabling collaboration across sectors when information and resources are limited constitute the capacity-building imperative (Bangkok Principle 4). This cannot remain dependent on ad hoc training or individual faculty enthusiasm. Disaster nursing competencies must be systematically integrated across undergraduate and graduate nursing curricula—not as optional electives but as core requirements. Field placements in disaster-affected communities or disaster-prone contexts should be required, not merely encouraged, providing students with experiential learning about risk assessment, participatory planning, and crisis operations. Cultivating disaster nursing specialists requires more than clinical skills. Interdisciplinary competence spanning public health, emergency management, urban planning, engineering, and social science becomes essential for effective collaboration. APNs leading disaster response must communicate effectively with structural engineers assessing building safety, urban planners redesigning evacuation routes, social workers addressing mental health, and community organizers mobilizing mutual aid networks. This interdisciplinary capacity requires intentional curricula, not osmosis—courses co-taught across disciplines, problem-based learning addressing complex scenarios requiring integration, and research collaborations modeling interdisciplinary practice.

8.7.5 First-Mile Co-Design and Co-Delivery: Institutionalizing Partnership

Establishing recurring health-emergency platforms at each administrative level—municipal, district, regional, national—to convene stakeholders for both slow-onset disasters like droughts and sudden-onset events like earthquakes (Bangkok Principle 5) institutionalizes the first-mile principle. These platforms cannot remain reactive, convening only when disasters occur. They must function continuously, meeting regularly to review risk assessments, update plans, conduct drills, and evaluate emerging threats. Regular engagement builds trust and familiarity that becomes operational capacity during crises when rapid coordination is essential.

Enabling nurses and APNs to propose cooperation from a lifestyle and health perspective—rather than merely responding to emergency management agendas—respects nursing's unique expertise in understanding how people actually live, what health needs emerge from daily practices, and what barriers prevent protective actions. Emergency managers understand logistics and command structures. Urban planners understand infrastructure and land use. Nurses understand how care responsibilities shape evacuation decisions, how chronic diseases require continuity of medication supply, and how cultural practices influence health behavior. Platforms that privilege emergency management perspectives while treating health as a support function waste nursing expertise. Effective platforms position nursing as equal partners whose perspectives actively shape strategy, not merely implementers of plans designed by others.

8.7.6 APN Leadership Functions: Policy Broker, Data Steward, Cross-Sector Convener

Advanced Practice Nurses operating at the intersection of clinical practice, community health, and institutional policy must function as policy brokers—translating clinical realities observed in field practice into policy recommendations, and translating policy decisions back into implementation guidance for frontline workers. When APNs observe systematic failures—evacuation plans incompatible with caregiving realities, medication supply chains breaking predictably during disasters, communication systems excluding non-dominant language speakers—they have a professional responsibility to escalate these observations to policy levels and advocate for systemic corrections. This brokerage function requires both clinical credibility to recognize problems and policy literacy to propose viable solutions.

APNs must also serve as data stewards—protecting consent, ensuring data quality, and advocating for equity in disaster health data flows. When vulnerable populations systematically lack data representation (undocumented migrants avoiding official systems, homebound elderly invisible to surveys), APNs must document these gaps and advocate for corrective data collection. When consent protocols inadequately protect privacy during emergencies, APNs must negotiate governance improvements. When data quality issues—missing variables, miscoded information, and sampling biases—undermine analysis reliability, APNs must intervene to improve data integrity.

Finally, APNs function as cross-sector conveners—enabling first-mile co-design across health, emergency management, engineering, telecommunications, and other partners. Disaster response requires coordination among sectors that normally operate independently with distinct cultures, vocabularies, and priorities. Health workers prioritize patient care; emergency managers prioritize operational efficiency;

engineers prioritize technical standards; telecommunications companies prioritize commercial viability. APNs who understand multiple sectors' perspectives and can translate across professional languages become essential integrators, convening partnerships that would otherwise fail due to miscommunication and misaligned incentives. With these science-to-action responsibilities articulated in alignment with international frameworks, the operational question becomes whether digital systems build trust, protect dignity, and reduce vulnerability—or amplify harm. This question brings us to open governance as the determinant of whether digital transformation serves disaster resilience or undermines it.

8.8 Open Governance: Trust as Infrastructure for Disaster Resilience

In disaster contexts, trust is not an abstract ethical value or desirable social outcome—it is operational infrastructure as essential as roads, communication networks, and medical supply chains. Without trust, early warnings are ignored despite accuracy because communities doubt the authorities' intentions. Shelters remain underutilized despite capacity because residents fear surveillance or exploitation. Rumors and misinformation dominate information flows because official sources lack credibility. Aid distribution becomes contested and violent because communities perceive unfairness in resource allocation. These trust failures directly translate into preventable casualties, prolonged suffering, and impaired recovery.

Open governance provides the structural mechanisms through which communities can observe, question, and genuinely co-own decisions about resources, data use, and trade-offs—transforming trust from an intangible social sentiment into measurable, cultivable infrastructure that directly impacts disaster outcomes. This requires explicit design across three nested layers: service delivery redesigned around lived experience, technical infrastructure embedding privacy and consent, and governance institutionalizing fairness and accountability as enforceable rules rather than aspirational principles.

8.8.1 Service Layer: Lived Experience as Design Foundation

Disaster health services must be designed around lived experience—shelter flow patterns, caregiving burdens, disability access requirements, language support needs—not merely institutional convenience or administrative efficiency. When shelter layouts require long walks between sleeping areas and bathrooms, elderly residents with mobility limitations face impossible choices between hydration and incontinence. When registration processes require documentation that displaced populations have lost, families remain without aid. When food distribution assumes nuclear families, extended family structures common in many Asian contexts face logistical barriers. These design failures are not mere inconveniences—they are equity failures that leave vulnerable populations underserved. Participatory service design processes engage affected communities in identifying requirements before facilities are built or systems deployed. Shelter design workshops where community representatives walk through mock layouts, identifying accessibility barriers. Food distribution simulations where families describe actual household compositions and cultural food practices. Communication system testing with non-dominant language speakers and low-literacy users. These participatory processes surface requirements that professionals consistently overlook, preventing costly redesigns after deployment failures.

8.8.2 Infrastructure Layer: Privacy, Consent, and Resilience by Design

Technical infrastructure for disaster data systems must embed privacy protection, consent management, and offline fallback capacity as fundamental architecture, not afterthoughts. Interoperable data flows connecting health systems, emergency management, and community organizations require role-based access controls specifying exactly what information each actor can view and modify. Spatial information networks mapping vulnerable populations must implement strong security measures to prevent unauthorized access while enabling rapid authorized response during emergencies. Offline fallback systems—paper backups, local data caches, and analog communication channels—ensure continued operation during power outages and network failures that inevitably accompany major disasters. Consent management becomes particularly complex during disasters when normal procedures may be impractical. Governance protocols must distinguish routine operations (requiring explicit opt-in consent), emergency operations (permitting broader information sharing under clearly defined triggers), and post-emergency transitions (returning to routine consent rules or deleting emergency-accessed data). Communities must participate in defining these consent rules, not merely be informed of expert-designed protocols. When communities trust that consent rules reflect their values and that violations will be detected and punished, participation in risk assessment and preparedness increases.

8.8.3 Governance Layer: Institutionalizing Fairness and Accountability

Institutionalizing fairness, transparency, and cultural adaptation as enforceable rules—including algorithmic accountability for AI-mediated triage or resource prioritization—prevents governance from remaining merely aspirational rhetoric. Multi-stakeholder governance committees with resident representation, independent audit authority, and genuine decision power can enforce fairness standards. When resource allocation algorithms systematically disadvantage specific populations, community representatives with audit access can detect and challenge these biases. When emergency protocols conflict with cultural practices, community members with co-decision authority can negotiate acceptable modifications.

Algorithmic accountability mechanisms become essential as AI systems increasingly mediate disaster decisions. Triage algorithms determining treatment priority, resource allocation models directing medical supply distribution, and evacuation routing systems calculating optimal paths all embed value judgments that may systematically disadvantage vulnerable populations. Algorithmic accountability requires explainability (decision rationales must be documentable and reviewable), contestability (communities can challenge outputs they believe are unfair), and correction mechanisms (when bias is demonstrated, algorithms must be modified or overridden). Multi-stakeholder governance, distributing decision rights among residents, clinicians, public health officials, emergency managers, technologists, and civil society organizations, prevents any single perspective from dominating. Residents bring irreplaceable knowledge about community values, actual living conditions, and informal social networks. Clinicians understand health needs and care feasibility. Public health officials assess population patterns and equity implications. Emergency managers coordinate logistics and interagency collaboration. Technologists design systems and analyze data. Civil society organizations represent marginalized groups and hold institutions accountable. Effective governance structures these diverse perspectives into decision processes where each is heard, conflicts are negotiated, and decisions reflect integrated judgment rather than single-sector dominance.

Trust grows when decisions are explainable and reversible—when communities can trace how inputs led to specific actions and how feedback influences subsequent iterations. Decision logs documenting why specific resource allocations occurred, what data informed decisions, and who made final judgments enable retrospective accountability. When communities understand decision rationales—even when disagreeing with outcomes—trust can be maintained. When decisions appear arbitrary or mysterious, trust collapses regardless of actual soundness. Reversibility means acknowledging mistakes and adjusting course when feedback reveals problems, rather than defending initial decisions despite evidence of harm. These governance principles become concrete and operational through digital transformation processes. Disaster nursing must lead digital transformation (DX) not merely as a technical system implementation but as an ethical and practical discipline determining whether technology serves resilience or undermines it.

8.9 Nursing DX in Disasters: Interoperability, Ethics, and Offline Resilience

Digital transformation in disaster nursing is fundamentally not mere digitization—converting paper records to electronic formats, replacing telephone communication with emails, or adding tablets to existing workflows. It is the comprehensive redesign of workflows, information flows, responsibility structures, and consent protocols so that information reaches where it can save lives without producing new forms of exclusion or surveillance. This distinction is critical: poorly designed digitization can actually reduce disaster resilience by creating single points of failure (digital systems that fail when power fails), excluding populations without digital access, and enabling surveillance that erodes trust. True nursing DX must be evaluated by its performance under stress conditions that inevitably accompany disasters: prolonged power outages, network infrastructure failures, overwhelming information volume, linguistic diversity barriers, misinformation storms, and severe workforce depletion. Systems that function well under normal conditions often catastrophically fail precisely when most needed—during the chaos of disaster response. Stress-testing DX systems through realistic scenarios before disasters strike becomes a patient safety imperative, not a nice-to-have enhancement.

8.9.1 Interoperability: Bridging Fragmented Systems

Interoperability matters vastly more than novelty or sophistication for disaster nursing systems. Cutting-edge AI analytics are operationally useless if they cannot communicate with public health databases, emergency medical services records, emergency operations centers, and community organization information systems. Nursing data must seamlessly bridge these disparate systems with clear role-based access rules and a minimal shared core dataset that all systems can exchange regardless of vendor or platform differences. Achieving this interoperability requires technical standardization (common data formats, shared communication protocols) but more fundamentally requires governance agreements specifying what information flows where, who can access it, for what purposes, and under what authorization. Technical standards enable information exchange; governance agreements ensure that the exchange serves legitimate purposes with appropriate safeguards. Pre-negotiating these governance agreements during peaceful times—rather than improvising during crises—prevents delays and conflicts when rapid information sharing becomes critical.

The minimal core dataset for disaster nursing must balance comprehensiveness and feasibility. Too minimal, and critical information for triage and resource allocation is missing. Too comprehensive, and systems become cumbersome, privacy-invasive, and difficult to maintain. Core elements typically include: demographic information enabling population-level analysis, location enabling spatial response coordination, health status markers for triage and resource prioritization, medication dependencies requiring continuity of supply, mobility limitations affecting evacuation feasibility, language/communication needs for effective information delivery, and emergency contacts for family reunification.

8.9.2 Multi-Source Sensing and Sensemaking: Big Data Integration

Building routine peacetime data pipelines that can rapidly ingest big data, social media streams (including Twitter/X), location information, community reports, sensor networks, and official surveillance systems enables rapid situational awareness when disasters strike (Minami, 2023). These systems cannot be designed and deployed during emergencies—they require sustained development, testing, and refinement during normal operations so that escalation to emergency mode is seamless. Social media monitoring provides early signals that official systems miss: residents posting about localized flooding before it appears in government sensors, concerns about rumors spreading that require rapid official response, and reports of specific needs (medications, infant formula, and disability equipment) enabling targeted supply distribution. However, social media data require sophisticated filtering to separate signals from noise, detect coordinated misinformation campaigns, and respect privacy—not all public social media posts are appropriate for official monitoring.

AI may assist triage and logistics—identifying patterns in massive data volumes that humans cannot process quickly enough, optimizing resource routing, or flagging high-priority cases for human review. However, nursing must retain accountable judgment and explainability rather than deferring to algorithmic outputs. When AI triage recommends deprioritizing specific patients, nurses must understand the rationale and possess the authority to override when clinical judgment or ethical principles demand it. Accountability cannot be outsourced to "the algorithm"—human professionals must remain responsible for consequences.

8.9.3 Multilingual and Low-Tech Communication by Design

Multilingual support and low-tech communication options must be designed into systems from inception, not retrofitted afterward when exclusions become undeniable. Pairing automated translation functions with human interpretation, plain-language rewriting of technical messages, and pictogram-first interfaces ensures that evacuation guidance, medical instructions, and consent processes are usable across linguistic diversity and literacy levels. Automated translation provides rapid scaling but makes errors that can be dangerous in medical contexts. Human interpreters provide accuracy but are resource-limited. Optimal systems combine both: automated translation for broad dissemination with human interpretation for critical communications requiring nuanced understanding.

Pictogram-first interface design—using universally recognizable symbols rather than text—improves usability for both low-literacy and non-native-language users. Evacuation route signs using arrows and human figures rather than text instructions. Medical equipment labeled with pictograms showing usage. Shelter facilities are marked with universally recognized symbols (bed, toilet, food, and medical care). While seemingly simple, pictogram design requires cultural sensitivity—symbols that seem universal may have culture-specific meanings that confuse or offend.

8.9.4 Telecom and Engineering Partnerships: Preparedness Infrastructure

Pre-negotiating agreements with private telecommunications companies for priority connectivity, rapid infrastructure restoration, and ethically governed location-based services—and testing these agreements through drills—prevents delays when disasters strike. Telecommunications companies understandably prioritize commercial operations and normal customer service. During disasters, these priorities may conflict with emergency response needs: allocating limited network capacity to government communications rather than commercial traffic, rapidly restoring damaged infrastructure in disaster zones rather than more profitable areas, and sharing location data to help locate isolated individuals despite privacy concerns. Preparedness agreements negotiated during peacetime establish protocols for these exceptional circumstances: what constitutes emergency activation, how priorities shift from commercial to emergency operations, what information sharing is authorized under what safeguards, how quickly restoration occurs, and how costs are covered. Testing these agreements through realistic drills reveals implementation challenges before actual disasters, when failures cost lives.

8.9.5 Design for Failure and for Rights: Offline Redundancy and Emergency Consent

Offline redundancy—paper workflows, local data caches, radio and analog communication channels—and emergency consent pathways constitute patient safety requirements, not optional enhancements. Every digital system should have documented procedures for continued operation when power fails, networks collapse, or digital infrastructure becomes inaccessible. Paper backup records, while cumbersome, remain readable when all electronics fail. Local data caches stored on field devices enable continued operation when network connectivity is lost. Radio and analog communication channels function when Internet-based systems fail. Emergency consent pathways recognizing that normal consent procedures may be impossible during disasters—unconscious patients requiring immediate treatment, displaced populations lacking documentation, chaotic conditions preventing detailed explanations—require pre-established protocols. These protocols must be clear about what emergency conditions justify modified consent procedures, what safeguards remain in effect even under emergencies, who has authority to invoke emergency procedures, and how return to normal consent occurs after situations stabilize.

APNs serving as on-scene integrators who keep governance obligations operational under stress conditions bridge the gap between ideal governance protocols and crisis reality. When normal committee structures cannot convene quickly enough, when documentation systems fail, or when ethical dilemmas require rapid resolution, APNs with governance training make field judgments preserving core principles while adapting to circumstances. This requires advance preparation—ethics training, governance authority, and institutional backing to make binding decisions under pressure. With disaster-ready DX specified for stress conditions rather than merely normal operations, the next imperative is treating inclusion not as an ethical aspiration but as a concrete safety requirement embedded in system design and operational protocols.

8.10 "Leaving No One Behind" in Disasters: Inclusion as a Safety Requirement

In disaster contexts, inequity functions as a hazard multiplier that transforms moderate events into catastrophes for vulnerable populations. The phrase "leaving no one behind"—drawn from the Sustainable Development Goals and increasingly invoked in disaster discourse—must be implemented through concrete design features and operational protocols, not merely aspirational statements in policy documents. Otherwise, it becomes empty rhetoric that fails precisely when vulnerability spikes during disasters, when marginalized populations face compounded harms while visible populations receive timely assistance. Disaster nursing, therefore, must treat inclusion as a safety requirement: if systems exclude any populations, the entire system is unsafe because exclusions create gaps where disease outbreak clusters, desperation breeds violence, and untreated injuries progress to preventable deaths. This is not merely an ethical principle but an epidemiological and operational reality. Infectious diseases spreading through excluded populations eventually affect all populations. Resource conflicts caused by unfair distribution threaten safety across all groups. Long-term recovery fails when some communities are rebuilt while others remain destroyed, breeding resentment and instability.

8.10.1 Design Communication for Diversity from Inception

Multilingual early warnings, plain-language message formats, trusted messenger networks, and cultural liaisons must be planned and resourced before crises occur, not improvised during response when time pressure and chaos make quality implementation impossible. Every disaster-prone region can enumerate its linguistic communities, assess literacy levels, and identify trusted community leaders. Translating core disaster messages into all local languages in advance—even if rarely needed—provides essential insurance. Training cultural liaisons who can interpret between emergency management and specific cultural communities—not merely translate words but explain concepts and mediate misunderstandings—builds capacity before crises. 10.2 Trusted messenger approaches recognize that official government sources may lack credibility with specific communities—migrants fearing deportation, undocumented workers avoiding authorities, and minority communities with historical grievances against government institutions. Partnering with community organizations, religious leaders, cultural associations, and informal networks that these communities trust enables information to flow through channels that official systems cannot reach.

8.10.2 Account for Caregiving Realities in All Plans

Evacuation and shelter logistics must integrate supports for infants, pregnancy, elder care, and disability assistance—not as special accommodations but as baseline requirements recognizing that caregiving defines daily reality for substantial populations. Evacuation plans assuming able-bodied individuals traveling independently fail for elderly caring for spouses with dementia, parents with young children, persons with mobility disabilities, and family structures where adult children care for elderly parents. Providing these supports—accessible transportation, disability-friendly shelters, childcare in emergency facilities, respite care for caregivers—determines whether vulnerable populations evacuate or remain in dangerous locations. Shelter designs must accommodate diverse caregiving needs: private family spaces (not just individual sleeping mats), equipment for infant care (cribs, formula preparation areas, and diaper changing facilities), accessible bathrooms and showers, medical equipment storage and charging, and quiet zones for people requiring reduced stimulation due to anxiety, autism, or trauma. These features are not luxuries—they are prerequisites for vulnerable populations to utilize shelters rather than remaining in collapsed buildings or flood zones deemed culturally or practically incompatible with their care needs.

8.10.3 Bridge the Digital Divide Proactively

Devices, connectivity, digital literacy training, and non-digital alternatives should be budgeted as DRR infrastructure investments, not left to individual responsibility. Disaster preparedness apps are useless for populations lacking smartphones. Early warning systems, depending on Internet access, exclude those without connectivity. Digital contact tracing fails when populations lack devices. These digital divides are not natural features but policy choices that can be addressed through intentional investment. Proactive strategies include: subsidized smartphone and data plans for low-income populations as public health infrastructure, public device charging and Internet access stations in community centers, simplified apps designed for low-end devices and limited connectivity, and mandatory non-digital alternatives (phone hotlines, radio broadcasts, and door-to-door outreach) ensuring zero dependence on digital access for critical services.

8.10.4 Protect Privacy and Dignity in Shelters

Shelter layout, hygiene facilities, gender-sensitive spaces, and confidential care pathways reduce harm, improve compliance with medical recommendations, and prevent exploitation and abuse. Crowded shelters with inadequate privacy, shared toilets without locks, and no separate spaces for vulnerable populations create environments where gender-based violence increases, disease transmission accelerates, and psychological trauma compounds. These harms are preventable through intentional design. Privacy protections include: partitioned family sleeping areas, lockable bathrooms, separate spaces for women and children feeling unsafe in mixed-gender areas, confidential medical consultation areas, and secure storage for personal belongings, preventing theft. Dignity-preserving features include: culturally appropriate hygiene facilities, religious accommodation (prayer spaces, ritual washing facilities), food respecting dietary restrictions and cultural preferences, and respect for traditional healing practices alongside conventional medicine.

8.10.5 Make Invisibility Visible Through Active Documentation

Routinely mapping who is missing from data and participation—undocumented migrants, homebound elderly, stigmatized populations (people with mental illness, HIV/AIDS, and substance use disorders), and geographically isolated communities—and redesigning outreach to reach these populations operationalizes inclusion. Exclusion often occurs not through malice but through system design defaulting to majority populations and failing to accommodate differences. Active documentation means explicitly recording gaps: evacuation plans reviewed by disability advocates documenting accessibility barriers, shelter designs tested by elderly users identifying mobility challenges, and communication materials assessed by non-native speakers identifying linguistic exclusions. When gaps are documented, they become visible problems demanding solutions rather than remaining unacknowledged and unaddressed. These concrete inclusion mechanisms can be operationalized only if we measure what actually matters for disaster resilience: not just physical losses and medical casualties but relational capacity to protect vulnerable populations through collective action sustained by trust and reciprocity.

8.11 Measuring What Matters: Empathetic Capital as Disaster Resilience Capacity

We propose empathetic capital as a measurable and cultivable community asset for disaster resilience: the aggregate capacity to recognize diverse needs, including those never explicitly articulated, translate understanding into decisions that feel fair even when imperfect, and sustain trust across linguistic, cultural, generational, and economic differences under uncertainty and resource scarcity. Empathetic capital complements conventional resilience metrics—infrastructure robustness, economic resources, medical system capacity—by capturing the relational infrastructure determining whether these material capacities actually function during crises when coordination and cooperation become survival requirements.

Traditional disaster risk metrics emphasize physical losses (deaths, injuries, and economic damage) and system capacities (hospital beds, emergency responders, and stockpiled supplies). While important, these metrics systematically miss relational factors consistently determining disaster outcomes. Communities with equivalent physical infrastructure and economic resources experience radically different disaster impacts based on social cohesion, institutional trust, and collective efficacy—factors that empathetic capital attempts to measure.

8.11.1 Empathetic Capital Growth Through Repeated Co-Design

Empathetic capital grows through repeated co-design cycles where participation patterns, reciprocity norms, perceived legitimacy of decisions, and feedback incorporation can be tracked longitudinally. Each participatory planning exercise, each community drill, each post-disaster review provides opportunities to build empathetic capital. Communities repeatedly engaged in co-design develop skills: articulating needs, understanding constraints, negotiating trade-offs, and resolving conflicts. Trust deepens through sustained engagement, demonstrating that institutions genuinely listen and incorporate community input. Measuring empathetic capital requires tracking process indicators: participation rates (who attends planning meetings), diversity of participation (are marginalized voices present and heard), quality of deliberation (are conflicts resolved or merely suppressed), institutional responsiveness (is feedback incorporated into decisions or ignored), and perceived legitimacy (do communities believe processes are fair even when outcomes disappoint). These indicators predict disaster outcomes—communities with higher empathetic capital evacuate more readily, cooperate more effectively during response, and recover more equitably.

Empathetic capital links directly to disaster outcomes through mechanisms that quantitative studies increasingly document. Higher trust reduces evacuation resistance—people comply with warnings when they trust information sources and believe authorities act in their interests rather than merely seeking control. Lower rumor spread occurs in communities with institutional trust and strong interpersonal networks, enabling rapid fact-checking. More equitable resource distribution happens when participatory governance enables affected populations to contest unfair allocations. Faster recovery occurs in communities with social cohesion, enabling collective reconstruction efforts rather than fragmented individual responses. Post-disaster studies consistently show that communities with strong pre-existing social networks, institutional trust, and participatory governance experience lower casualties, faster evacuation, more effective mutual aid, less conflict over resources, and more equitable recovery. These outcomes are not random variation but direct consequences of empathetic capital that can be deliberately cultivated through sustained institutional investment in participatory governance, community engagement, and trust-building before disasters strike.

8.11.2 Education as Empathetic Capital Investment

Education systems integrating ethnography, participatory design, GIS literacy, and disaster ethics as core nursing competencies represent a strategic investment in empathetic capital. Nurses trained only in clinical protocols and efficiency metrics cannot build empathetic capital—they lack methodological tools for deep listening, cultural understanding, participatory engagement, and ethical deliberation. Curricular reform integrating these capabilities produces graduates equipped to function as empathetic capital builders rather than merely technical service providers.

This educational investment requires reshaping not just content but pedagogy. Participatory methods cannot be learned from lectures—they require experiential practice through community engagement, participatory action research projects, ethnographic fieldwork, and sustained relationship-building with communities different from students' backgrounds. Disaster ethics cannot be reduced to case studies—it requires facilitated deliberation, practicing how to make principled decisions under uncertainty with conflicting values and insufficient information.

8.11.3 Governance-Ready Metrics Beyond Clinical Outcomes

Governance-ready metrics must accompany conventional clinical metrics, capturing not just medical outcomes but who was reached by services, who participated meaningfully in decisions, who benefited equitably from resource distribution, and who remained at risk despite interventions. Medical success (lives saved, injuries treated) provides a necessary but insufficient assessment of disaster nursing performance. If success was concentrated among privileged populations while vulnerable groups remained underserved, the system failed regardless of aggregate medical outcomes. Equity-sensitive metrics disaggregate outcomes by demographics (age, gender, ethnicity, disability status, and economic class), geography (urban versus rural, proximity to services), and vulnerability status (pre-existing health conditions, social isolation, and language barriers). Comparing outcomes across these categories reveals whether systems serve all equitably or systematically advantage some while disadvantaging others. When disparities are documented, they become visible problems demanding governance responses rather than remaining implicit and unaddressed.

In the digital age, the strongest indicator of disaster readiness is not data volume accumulated in databases or algorithmic sophistication of analytical systems but the community's demonstrated capacity to act together effectively—coordinating rapid response, making fair decisions under pressure, maintaining trust across differences, and learning continuously from both successes and failures. This collective capacity, what we term empathetic capital, determines whether technical systems become operational assets or merely expensive infrastructure that fails when most needed because people refuse to use systems they distrust. These conceptual elements—disaster nursing as integrative discipline, spatial computing as consensus infrastructure, culture-led development as values compass, empathy translation as methodological craft, Jimoto as first-mile practice site, science-to-action as international framework alignment, open governance as trust infrastructure, disaster-ready DX as resilience requirement, inclusion as safety standard, and empathetic capital as resilience asset—converge in a single conclusion articulating disaster nursing's role in the digital age.

8.12 Conclusion: Transformative Community Health Nursing as Disaster Nursing and Community Resilience

This volume has argued systematically that transformative community health nursing is fundamentally inseparable from disaster resilience in the digital age. Planetary health disruption, syndemic risks, NATECH disasters, and complex cascading hazards require nursing to operate as a systems discipline integrating data with culture, technology with ethics, evidence with narrative, and rapid action with community ownership. The conventional boundaries separating emergency nursing, public health nursing, and community health nursing have become obsolete—disaster resilience requires integration across this spectrum. Our central proposition is not merely new terminology or conceptual reframing but a practical reorientation: disaster nursing must adopt a science-to-action posture aligned with the Sendai Framework and Bangkok Principles—where interventions are co-designed and co-delivered with communities, governance is explicit and enforceable, and the most vulnerable populations are served first rather than last or never. This reorientation challenges deeply embedded professional norms valuing expert autonomy, top-down authority, and protocol compliance over participatory partnership, cultural adaptation, and community ownership.

Acknowledgments The author thanks Seiko Iimura (research assistant, Kobe City College of Nursing) for her indispensable editorial and logistical support throughout the preparation of this concluding chapter. Generative AI tools assisted with structuring and language refinement; all content was critically reviewed, revised, and approved by the author. This chapter draws on insights shared by community partners, local governments, and frontline nursing practitioners across Japan, whose collective wisdom underpins the concept of Jimoto Sousei Nursing. The author is grateful to all contributors to this volume whose work made the synthesis presented here possible. Special thanks are due to Prof. Hiroshi Okumura for his foundational philosophy of Open Governance and Challenge Open Governance (COG), for his generous guidance throughout the development of this volume, and for his ongoing work in developing practical tools for civic participation and community resilience.

Author Contributions Conceptualization and synthesis: Sakiko Kanbara. Writing—original draft: Sakiko Kanbara. Writing—review and editing: Sakiko Kanbara; editorial and linguistic assistance provided by a research assistant (Seiko Iimura). Literature search, reference management, and manuscript preparation: research assistant (Seiko Iimura). AI-assisted drafting: Generative AI tools were used to support structuring, synthesis, and language refinement under the supervision of Sakiko Kanbara.

Appendices: Handout-Ready Templates

Templates can be provided as separate files or online supplements. Suggested components:

Appendix A: Spatialization Checklist (GIS/Map Minimum Requirements)

- Define purpose (dialogue, planning, triage) and avoid surveillance framing.
- Minimum layers: people (aggregated), places (clinics/shelters), access (routes/barriers/time), hazards, and resources (volunteers/supplies).
- Accessibility: produce a printed map packet and a simple legend; prepare "no smartphone" pathways.
- Update rhythm: who updates what, how often, and how changes are communicated offline.
- Safety: do not publish granular data that could expose individuals; apply redaction where needed.
- Use in meetings: put the map on the table; let residents correct it ("ground-truthing").

Appendix B: Community Scoping Sheet (Fill-In Template)

Community (place)	__
Core purpose (for whom?)	__
Primary risks (hazards + everyday disasters)	__
Stakeholders (who is usually "at the table")	__
Absent/ 'silent" groups (who is missing?)	__
Key places (clinics, shelters, lifelines, gathering points)	__
Cultural values (what counts as "good" locally)	__
Capacity constraints (people, time, budget, trust)	__
90-day pilot boundary (what we will test, and what we will not)	__
Next meeting (date + facilitator + outputs to bring)	__

Appendix C. Empathy Preservation Interview Guide

- Opening (everyday life): "Walk me through a normal day. Where do care and health decisions happen?"
- Crisis memory: "In the last disaster/health crisis, what became hardest to maintain (water, food, sleep, privacy, care work)?"
- Hidden friction: "What did you hesitate to say or ask for? Why?" (Listen for silence and indirect cues.)
- Digital divide: "When information is sent by smartphone or online, what becomes easier/harder for you or your family?"
- Mutual aid: "Who helped you first? Who was left out? What made help possible or impossible?"
- Cultural "good": "What would a 'good' response look like in this community? What would feel unacceptable?"

- Closing (give-back): "If we change one thing in the next 90 days, what should it be? How should we report back to you?"
- Consent check: confirm permission for note-taking/recording; explain routine vs emergency use; confirm right to withdraw.

References

Miyamae, S., Kanbara, S., Owaza W., Fujii, M., Nakajima M., Yamamoto, A., Minami, H., (2023). Identifying research topics for disaster nursing science from the perspective of nursing researchers using the Delphi method. Japan Society of Disaster Nursing, 25 (2) (In Japanese).

Science Council of Japan (SCJ). (2020). *Proposal on promoting collaboration between nursing science and society to realize "local community creation" (Jimoto Sousei)*. Science Council of Japan. (In Japanese).

Shaw, R. (2020). Thirty years of science, technology, and academia in disaster risk reduction and emerging responsibilities. *International Journal of Disaster Risk Science, 11*(4), 414–425. https://doi.org/10.1007/s13753-020-00264-z

United Nations (UN). (2015). *Sendai framework for disaster risk reduction 2015–2030*. United Nations Office for Disaster Risk Reduction.

United Nations Office for Disaster Risk Reduction (UNDRR), & World Health Organization (WHO). (2016). *Bangkok Principles for the implementation of the health aspects of the Sendai framework for disaster risk reduction 2015–2030*. UNDRR & WHO.

GPSR Compliance

The European Union's (EU) General Product Safety Regulation (GPSR) is a set of rules that requires consumer products to be safe and our obligations to ensure this.

If you have any concerns about our products, you can contact us on ProductSafety@springernature.com

In case Publisher is established outside the EU, the EU authorized representative is:

Springer Nature Customer Service Center GmbH
Europaplatz 3
69115 Heidelberg, Germany

Batch number: 10800012

Printed by Printforce, the Netherlands